WWW.ZODIACSERVICES.NET

Presents

DO IT YOURSELF – MAHA REMEDY POOJAS!

A SIMPLE HANDBOOK OF HINDU REMEDY WORSHIP POOJAS & PARIGARAMS

A SIMPLE GUIDE TO HINDU MAHA PARIGARA POOJAS!

Life Grows With Us!

SIMPLE & EASY WAY TO UNDERSTAND THE BASICS OF HINDU REMEDY POOJA AND WORSHIP EASILY IN SUMMARY AND KEY CONCEPTS WITH EFFECTIVE CHAPTERS & TOPICS OF MANTRAS AND ASHTOTRAMS!

By

G.R. Narasimhan

Welcome to Zodiac Services remedy poojas in brief with effective topics and additional special mantars to achieve any goal with divine blessings!

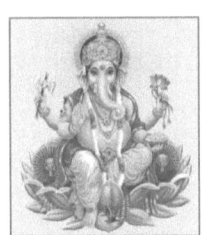

I0425599

ALSO INCLUDES NAVARATHRI POOJA / LAGU HOMAM/YAGNA

GOOD LUCK TO ACHIEVE SUCCESS BY REMEDY POOJAS!

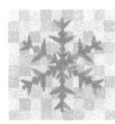

Zodiac Services, Chennai, India

Get more contact details and numbers from:

www.zodiacservices.net [or] mail to info@zodiacservices.net

Ordering Information for hardcopies:

Quantity sales – Special discounts are available on quantity purchases by corporations, associations and others. For details, contact the author at the address above.

JULY 2019 – First Edition

Released and Published in Amazon India

ABOUT THE AUTHOR

G.R. Narasimhan – Sr. Consultant for technology and business under **Zodiac Services Chennai** which was started in 2010 to serve the people in alternative beliefs/therapies like astrological predictions, prayers, remedies, prasanam (divine words) and vedic guidance for short- or long-term problems, vaastu, numerology, gem stones, yantras, mantras or rituals (related areas), yoga, meditation, counseling and alternative therapies consulting. Business & education, soft skills/software/electronics & communication training & promotion, web designing, career counseling and Internet & social media marketing are additionally served. Assisting the entrepreneurship business for the above mentioned areas to serve better for the clients, **G.R. Narasimhan** also the author of few e-books called "A Simple guide to Vedic Astrology," "Inverted Universal Meditation & Engineering," "Secrets of Equity Stocks to make Millions," "Symbolic Meditation & Developing ESP", "MBA Basics in 24 Hours" and many other (are already available in Amazon) having extended experience in IT + Management areas developed website and online marketing using different business strategies and continue the service very well to extend further including this "A Simple Guide to Hindu Remedy Poojas" concepts specifically based on the effective topics applied overall in the remedy pooja cycle in single shot. With the continuous extraordinary ability and skills in research and experience, he is able to explain and train/assist others with extended support and guidance by counseling/consulting effectively.

Great thanks and good luck for everyone reading this book on "A Simple Guide to Hindu Remedy Poojas" with almost all the areas of basic success in achieving goals / growth individually or as a group. For any queries and feedback, you can contact directly via email to info@zodiacservices.net, info@astroservices.in or astronara@gmail.com.

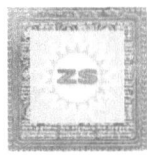

CONTENTS

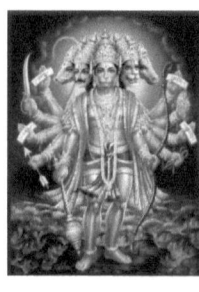

INTRODUCTION

Poojas and Remedies are certain belief system of angelic invocation & worship to attain siddhi or some goals to be achieved in life with the help of divine and blessings from the almighty. As per Hindu traditional belief systems; there are so many angelic presences like Lord Ganapathy, Lord Hanuman, Lord Shiva, Lord Vishnu, Lakshmi Devi, Gowri Devi, Saraswathi Devi and so on. Every angelic presence having a particular power to help the people in certain ways; for example if Goddess Saraswathi is worshiped, then people would get good education. Similarly for getting prosperity the Goddess Lakshmi to be worshiped.

Worship or prayers to attain certain siddhis/ powers, or achieving some goals in life like good job/ business, education, marriage, travel etc; could be in many ways as follows.

- Simple prayers by chanting the particular angelic name and saying your wish. (can be done anywhere)
- By chanting gayatri mantras/ moola mantras or chanting 108 or 1008 names of a particular devta or angelic presence. (can be done anywhere)
- Offering flowers, fruits and some holy food like sweet pongal, rice etc at temple or home and do some mantras chanting. (Poojas)
- Doing poojas with picture or kalasam (vessel containing holy water) by chanting mantras.
- Yagam or Yagnam – holy fire ritual performed to invoke angelic presence in fire and do the worship by offering ghee and holy herbals etc. (Havan/ Yagnam)
- Requesting others to do the above prayers on behalf of you. (Guru)

Gayatri mantra is the first and best chanting method of invoking angelic presence. Each presence has its own gayatri mantra and that has the most power of invocation. Next one is moola mantra of that particular god or goddess. This with some beeja mantras can give expected results as per Hindu vedic belief system. Again ashtotram (108 names) or

Sahasra-namam (1000/1008 names) of that particular angel or god would give the best result for prayers and answered.

Among all the mantra meditation practices in the world, after "Om" beejam chanting power, the Gayatri mantra plays vital role to attain spiritual & material growth. Gayatri Devi is an angel who owns the mantra and able to help everyone who follows this mantra and gives all the benefits in life. <u>Gayatri Mantra or Beejam produces more than one lakh sound waves per second</u>. This is most powerful hymn or sound wave in the world. The combination of sound or sound waves of this mantra is claimed capable of developing specific spiritual abilities.

<u>Material and Physical Benefits of this are:</u>
Aura cleansing & chakra balancing, Bestows attractive personality, develops the power of speech, removes poverty and insufficiency, forms a protective layer around the person, wards off dire influences, unfavorable circumstances and dangerous situations, automates spiritual & emotional balances, The beeja mantras in the mantra activates physical acupressure points, The vibrations while chanting spread in the atmosphere, attract similar positive atoms and return to its origin (the person who is chanting) filling him with this positive energy. Regular chanting keeps the person and his family always (with)/ in prosperity, abundance and wealthy status.

<u>The Gayatri Mantra is:</u>
Aum Bhuhr Bhuvah Suvah| Tat Savituh Varenyam|Bhargo Devasya Dhimahi| Dhiyo yo Nah Prachodayat|

<u>The meaning is</u>: "God is dear & close to me like my own breath, He is the dispeller of my pains and giver of happiness. I meditate on the supremely adorable Light of the Divine Creator / Almighty that it may inspire my thought and understanding forever!"

<u>The following qualities develop</u>: Love, Bravery, Wellbeing, Wealth, Brilliance, Immunity, Devotion Intellect, Controlling Senses, Attracts life force, Awakening, Courageous, Wisdom, Whole being cleansing! Etc.

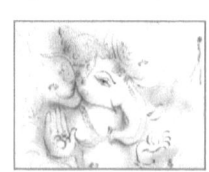

s many people wanted to do remedy pooja or parigaram; they depend n some people or Guru to perform the same for them with desired angalpam (intentions); sometimes they do not get. To help these eople or the people who wants to perform their own remedy; this book vould certainly help mainly for <u>Kalathra dhosham, Mangalya dhosham, hevvai (Angaraga) dhosham/ Kala Sarpa dhosham/ Bad karmic effect emoval etc. As of now it gave 100% good results for everone. I ersonally learned from my Guruji and performed this for many people. Vithout keeping it with me; I would like to release as a book for others.</u>

or all prayers to get good job, marriage, property, children, travel, usiness growth, health and longevity or removal of cursing in family or nunglik (angaraga dhosham), Kalasarpa dhosham (naga dhosham), three sabam and other blockages in horoscope etc; this pooja rocedure given in the book will be very useful and can be performed by ourself.

his book is guiding everyone who believes in Hinduism and prayers or oojas worship to do certain practices for different god or goddesses / ngelic presence to achieve all said benefits above. The chapters are xplaining how to do the poojas for many divine powers and which are nandatory / optional.

he advantages of remedy poojas/rituals are:

- The divine presence always protects us from any danger/trouble and misfortune.
- Shows us right path and guidance by intuition in all the matters.
- Improves wealth, stress relief and no bad influence of people.
- Blocks or removes any evil presence or evil eye attack in our mind, body or aura.
- Cleanses mentally and gives more strength and will power.
- Improves the soul radiation better to achieve more.
- Avoids bad companions automatically and safe guard us.
- Success in everyday life, career, family and travel etc.

- Cures many diseases automatically by divine blessing and keeps us healthy.
- Gives more power of making decision, brave and keeps rejuvenated.
- Appears in dream and teach us sometimes new mantras, methods and opportunities.
- Listen to our prayers and fulfils as per universal laws/attraction & more!

Nowadays most of the people are living in flats/apartment buildings or in rental houses are unable to perform yagam/yagnam due to space constraints or fire alarms/ association rules etc. But these poojas given in this can be performed easily to get full blessings anywhere in a small space or in pooja room by yourself or with the help of guruji/pandit.

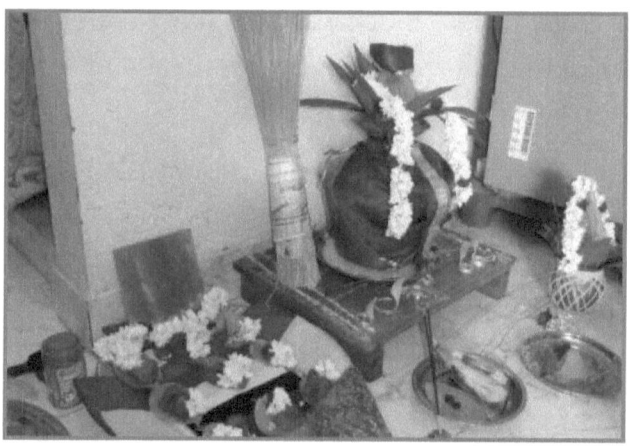

Before and after pooja photos (sample)

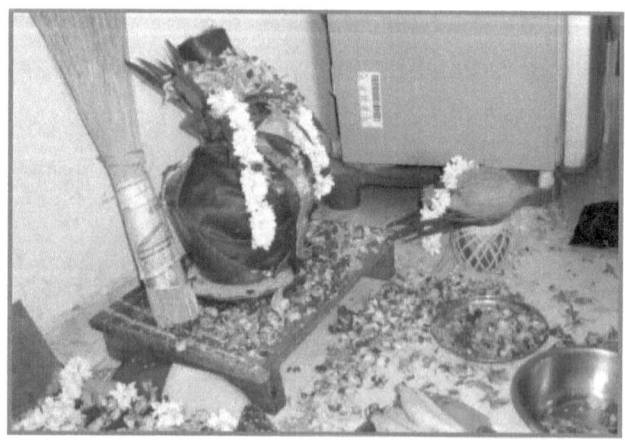

Wish you Good Luck!

Important Notes:

- Lord Ganapathy pooja & Hanuman pooja & Navagraga pooja will remove any navagraga dhosham/ragu-ketu or sani in general. Gives will power, physical power, emotional & spiritual balance.

- For mainly kalathira/ maangalya shosham – all Devi poojas are best. Here it has Lakshmi, Varahi, Gowri, Durga, Saraswathi, Lalitha, & Balambika.

- The above Devi poojas can be called as "Saptha Kaali Pooja" (7 Devis). Powerful to remove any obstacles as per vedic remedies.

- Also 7 Devis' pooja can be performed in Navarathri time as mainly we do Lakshmi, Durga and Saraswathi during the festival time.

- Nagaraja swami pooja is useful to remove Kala sarpam/ Naga dhosham including ragu-ketu negative effect. Also removes poison from aura field and energy field.

- Subramanya swami pooja is mainly for Mars negative effect, called Manglik – angaraga / chevvai dhosham. Also for fame, power, courageness, stops enemies at distance, job or career growth and so on.

- Though this entire pooja is bit difficult to do in one shot; it will be easy if you read and understand fully and practice.

- Mantras of Sanskrit words are given in English directly; though the words are difficult to pronounce, you can chant couple of times first to get into that and then do. Don't worry about wrong pronounciation. Because, more than chanting; the bakthi and your intention is very important here. If you believe, always divine blessings for all!

CHAPTER 1 – INITIAL / BASIC SETUP FOR THE POOJAS!

- Before starting the remedy pooja, you must clean the place. Sprinkle water and rub with cloth or mob the place.
- Then put some rangoli/ kolam if possible or just sprinkle chandan/sandal little. Keep one or two kalasam vessel ready as shown in the above picture.
- For Offerings, keep some fruits like banana, orange, apple etc whatever possible. Also if betel leaves and nut little (if possible).
- One or two coconuts required to keep on kalasams/vessels which can be filled with water and add some chandan powder in it little and some clove or krambu/ cardamom or edible camphor (anyone is available) in it for making it holy water.
- Only one kalasam vessel is enough for main pooja; but we can keep Varuna kalasam and Navagraga kalasam separately as shown in the above picture.
- Make arrangements as shown in the picture approximately.
- Keep holy bell and a small cup (one or two) of water with spoon.
- Dhoop or Ghee lamp also advisable for showing aarthi.
- Flowers to decorate and do archana (name chanting) for devatas or angelic presence are important. You can buy as per your choice. (Jasmine/ Rose/ Tulsi/Bilva or any auspicious flowers etc)
- If possible keep one small idol of Ganesh or Make it with turmeric (yellow powder). Or keep a small picture of Ganesh [optional]
- Just keep holy grass or dharpam grass along with. Pavitram can be made and wear in the ring finger during pooja. [optional]
- Can decorate kalasam with silk cloth or ordinary cloth and keep mango tree leaves (or betel leaves instead of mango tree leaves) on that and then coconut. Keep chandan and kumkum on kalasam and coconut and decorate as shown.
- Keep yourself clean after bathing and then put some chandan/kumkum as per your wish on the forehead.
- If available make yellow rice, by mixing yellow powder with rice for archana or just for sangalpam. But no issues; only flowers are also enough.

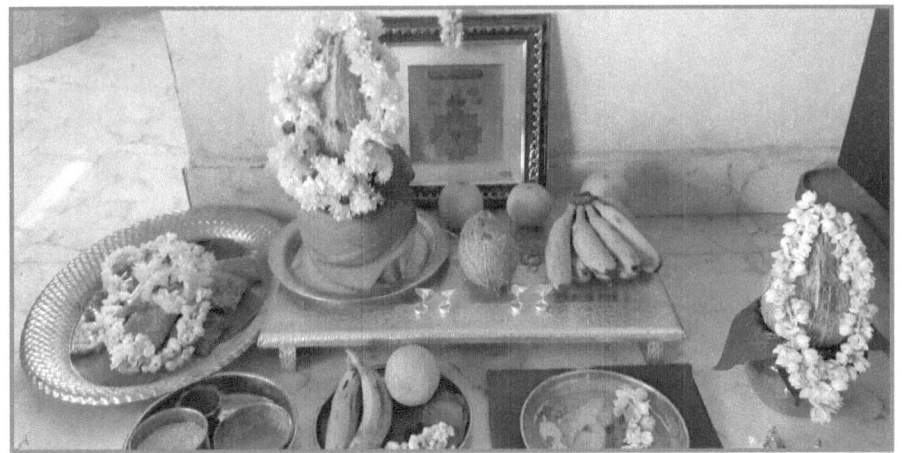

Check the above picture for another pooja setup:

- Middle vessel is main kalasam.
- Right side vessel is varuna kalasam. [optional]
- Left side tray has Nava-dhanyam for Navagraga pooja. You can keep another kalasam also for the same [optional]
- Behind the main kalasam, there is a Sri chakra/yantra for pooja (common for all devatas) – [optional]
- Flowers, fruits, yellow ganesh, akshatha-yellow rice, kumkum, chandan etc shown. Below picture shows after pooja:

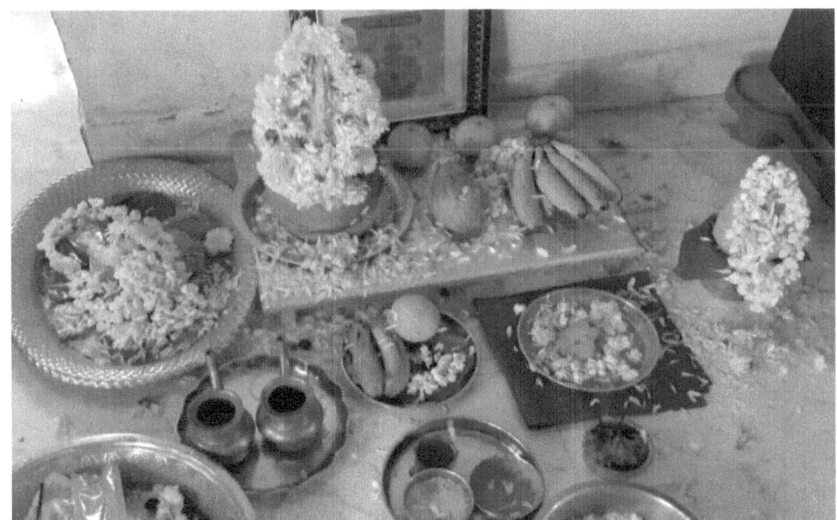

- Start the pooja with peace of mind and ablution. Once all the items are ready as per your wish, you can start the remedy pooja with sangalpam next. Sit infront of kalasam.

CHAPTER 2 –MAIN SANGALPAM/PURPOSE (INTENTIONS)

Sangalpam is simply to say what our main request is or what to achieve with the help of poojas or prayers. It is just like other prayers to initially say the things which you would like to achieve. Here most of the veda sastras are performing in Sanskrit language. This book gives entire pooja in English only including Sanskrit words in English. But you can also say in Hindi/ Telugu or Tamil or in any other language as per your wish. Mainly you have to be very clear with your prayer request. Before starting the sangalpam, keep pure water in a small container and consume it by pouring little in right hand 3 times by saying; ...

- Om Achudhaya Namaha
- Om Ananthaya Namaha
- Om Govindaya Namaha

Keep some flowers [and yellow rice/holy rice if possible] in your right hand and close it. Then start sangalpam/prayer intention.

Sangalpam in English:

OM – MAHA GANAPATHIYE NAMAHA:

OM - [Today as on DD/MM/YYYY][Time], [I am performing this remedy pooja for myself and family members to have good health, wealth, luck, prosperity, abundance, career growth, marriage, good children, education, longevity, good relationship, love and affection with family members and others, peace of mind, stress-free life, travel opportunities, safety], [spiritual, emotional, physical, energy & aura cleansing; balancing and strengthening], [removal of cursing from other sources, ancestors, divine beings, enemies, other people], [removal of negativity from others, karmas], [curing diseases, settlements, paying loans],[protection from disasters, hazards, enemies],[removal of munglik-angaraga dhosham, kala sarpa dhosham, kalathira dhosham, maangalya dhosham, family karmas],[removal of bad planetary effects (Navagraga dhosham), pancha boodha balancing] ....and so on.

Note: You can add or remove any request as per your wish along with this sangalpam/ intention/ desires of prayer.

Sangalpam in Sanskrit:

It has many types; but a simple one is recommended here

OM – MAHA GANAPATHIYE NAMAHA: OM Shube' shobane' Suba Muhurthe' aaditya brahmana ha: Dhvithiya prapthe' shwedha varaha kalpe' vaivas-va manvanthare' kaliyuge, pradhama paathe' jambudhrewe' baratha varushe, baratha kande [for other countries except india use the word 'rudhra kande' instead of 'baratha kande'] sahapthe' meroho dhakshine paaswe' asmin varthamane, viva karige, prabavathi shashti; samhasraanam asye', Uthirayane from months Sankranthi to Mithunam….) or Dhakshinayane' (from months Katagam to Dhanur maasam….), maha rudhu, maha maasa [mention month name here….], pakshow' ('Krishna paksha' for waning moon…'Sukla paksha' for waxing moon….] suba-thitha vasaraha ….(mention day name here…[Sunday-banu vasaraha, Monday-Indhu vasaraha, Tuesday-Mangala vasaraha, Wed-Soumya Varsaraha, Thu-Guru Vasaraha, Fri- Brigu Vasaraha….] Nakshatra …[mention today's star name here….like aswini, barani etc …else just leave], Sri bagavath lagna sreeman Narayana/ Parameswara preethyartham …[your name, gothram, star, raasi or moon sign followed by family members name and their stars, rasi, gothram etc].

Note: Refer panchang for star, day, rudhu, etc…After mentioning the above details, now intention the following.

Sarva shema, dhairya, veerya, vijaya, aayur aarokya, iswarya anugraga sidhirastham. Viyapara uthyoga anugraga sidhirastham, dhega bala, mano bala, janma bala, sareera bala anugraga sidhirastham, sarva devatha anugraga sidhirastham, ashta lakshmi kadaksha; ashta iswarya anugraga sidhirastham, prayana kaala sarva anugoola sidhirastham.

Kudumba shaba, deiva shaba, bramhna shaba, Gow shaba, sthree shaba, rishi shaba, deva shaba, sarva shaba, sharva dhosha nivarthi praya-chidartham. Sarva dushta devatha sanchara dhosha nivarthi, sarva chatru baya dhosha nivathihi, chatru drishti prayoga, dhushta sakthi prayoga, maandriga prayoga dhosha nivathihi.

Mangalya dhosha, kalathira dhosha, kaalasarpa dhosha, angaraga dhosha nivarthihi, jaadhaga pala sarva aadhitya dhi Navagraga dhosha nivarthi praya chithartham, parambara dhosha nivathihi, sarva jadhaga dhosha nivarthihi…aaramba kaala sangalpa pragaarenaha sarva praya chithartha …maha parhikara poojaam asya karishye']…… put the flowers/yellow rice aside!

Note: You can add or remove any request as per your wish along with this sangalpam/ intention/ desires of prayer.

If you do not know sangalpam in sanskrit, please do it in your language.No issues.

Sangalpam can be performed by keeping the yellow rice [rice mixed with turmeric] and little flower in hand. Once sangalpam done, just put it aside. Then we have to start Ganapathy pooja!

CHAPTER 3 – LORD GANESH POOJA

Before starting of any pooja or worship; Lord Ganesh pooja is mandatory as he is the primary deity who assists in our pooja / worship from sangalpam (intention) to end of the pooja. He himself basically acts as a protector and primary angel or higher self to give power and knowledge to attain any siddhi.

Simply gayatri manthra with some moola mantras for Lord Ganesh (Ganapathy) can be chanted along with the following 16 names are enough with offering some bananas or any fruit/ milk or sweets etc! Put flowers or kumkum or akshadha (yellow rice) for each chanting infront of Ganesh. Keep picture or idol, bell, dhoop, chandan, kumkum, fruits, flowers etc as per your wish!

Put some yellow rice with flowers / only flowers and say "Om Maha Ganapathi devatham aavagayami" – 1 time [means invoking lord ganesh in holy water and idol or picture], [or]

Om Ganapathiye nhama : aasanam samar-payaami, pathayae : paathyam Smar-payaami, hasthayoa arkkiyam samar-payaami, aachama-niiyam...samar-payaami. Sthaapa-yaami, Snaanam aachama-neeyam samar-payaami, vasthram, aaparanaam. upaviitham akshatham samarpayaami, kanhtham samarpayaami, kungkumam samarpayaami....

[then...1 time all mantras below...]

Ganapathy Gayatri Mantra

- *Om yega dhandaya vidmahe vakra thundaya dheemahi dhanno dhandi prachodayat |*

Ganapathy Moola Mantras

- **Om shreem hreem kleem kloumgam ganapathaye; Varavarada sarva janamme vasamaanaya swaha :**

- **Om ganesa runam siddhi varenyam hoom namaha bhat swaha :**

- **Om ganesarunam siddhi varenyam hoom namaha bhat swaha :**

- **Om vakra thundaya hoom |**

- **Om hreem kreem hreem maha ganapathaye namaha :**

<u>**Note**</u>: There are many other moola mantras are also available. Above mantras are enough for simple pooja.

<u>Shree Vinayaka Shodasa Namavali (16 names)</u>

<u>Chant all the below mantras after chanting gayatri and moola mantras. Put flowers on Ganesh.</u>

- Om- sumukaya -namaha
- Om- yegadanthaya -namaha
- Om- kabilaya -namaha
- Om- gajakarnakaya -namaha
- Om- lambodaraya -namaha
- Om- vikadaya -namaha

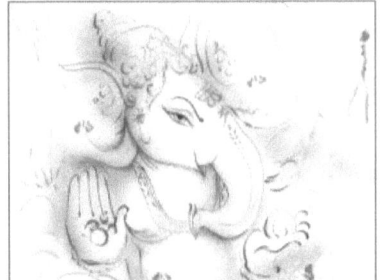

- Om- vignarajaya -namaha
- Om- ganadhi paya -namaha
- Om- dooma kedave -namaha
- Om- ganadh - yekshaya -namaha
- Om- balachandraya -namaha
- Om- gajananaya -namaha
- Om- vakra thundaya -namaha
- Om- soorpakarnaya -namaha
- Om- herambaya -namaha
- Om- skandha-poorvajaya –namaha

Om- maha ganapathaye –namaha :

Note: After chanting above mantras, ring the bell and show the dhoop for Lord Ganesh. Then offer fruits or milk/ sweets to him. We can also light up ghee lamp or sesame oil lamp if required! [This can be done after finishing below ashtothram also]

LORD GANESH ASHTOTHRAM

We can also chant the following ashtothram (108 names) for Lord Ganesh to extend the primary pooja which will be more helpful to get additional blessings! Follow the same procedures as said above. Do in main kalasam vessel. Put flowers [or yellow holy rice]

Om- vinayagaya -namaha

Om-vignarajaya-namaha

Om-gowri puthraya-namaha

Om-ganesh waraya-namaha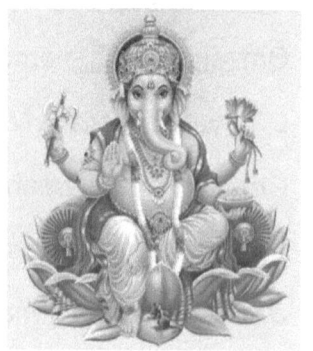

Om-skandha grajaya-namaha

Om-avya yaaya-namaha

Om-boodhaya-namaha

Om-dakshaya-namaha

Om-adyakshaya-namaha

Om-dvijapriya-namaha - 10

Om-agni karpachide-namaha

Om-indra shree pradaya-namaha

Om-vaani pradhaya-namaha

Om-avyaya-namaha

Om-sarvasiddhi pradaya-namaha

Om-sarva dhanayaya-namaha

Om-sarva priyaya-namaha

Om-sarva thmakaya-namaha

Om-srushti karthre-namaha

Om-devaya-namaha - 20

Om-anegarchithaya-namaha

Om-sivaya-namaha

Om-suddhaya-namaha

Om-budhipriyaya-namaha

Om-sandhaya-namaha

Om-brahma charine-namaha

Om-gajananaya-namaha

Om-dvai mathreyaya-namaha

Om-munis thuthyaya-namaha

Om-baktha vigna vinasanaya-namaha - 30

Om-yega dandaya-namaha

Om-chatur bahuve-namaha

Om-chaturaya-namaha

Om-sakthi samyuthaya-namaha

Om-lambodaraya-namaha

Om-soorpa karnaya-namaha

Om-haraye-namaha

Om-brahma viduthamaya-namaha

Om-kaalaya-namaha

Om-graha padaye-namaha - 40

Om-kamine-namaha

Om-soma-sooryagni-namaha

Om-lochanaya-namaha

Om-pasangu sadharaya-namaha

Om-sandaya-namaha

Om-gunadheethaya-namaha

Om-niranjanaya-namaha

Om-agal makshaya-namaha

Om-svayam siddhaya-namaha

Om-siddhar chita padam bujaya-namaha - 50

Om-beeja poora pala sakthaya-namaha

Om-varadhaya-namaha

Om-sasvathaya-namaha

Om-kruthinae-namaha

Om-dvijapriyaya-namaha

Om-veedhabayaya-namaha

Om-gathinae-namaha

Om-chakrinae-namaha

Om-ikshsusapathruthe-namaha

Om-shreedaraya-namaha - 60

Om-ajaya-namaha

Om-uthpalakaraya-namaha

Om-shreepadaye-namaha

Om-sathu dihark shithaya-namaha

Om-kulathri bethre-namaha

Om-jatilaya-namaha

Om-kalikalmashanasanaya-namaha

Om-chandrasoodamanaye-namaha

Om-kaandhaya-namaha

Om-papaharinae-namaha - 70

Om-samahithaya-namaha

Om-aasrithaya-namaha

Om-shreekaaraya-namaha

Om-sowmyaya-namaha

Om-bhaktha vanjitha thayakaya-namaha

Om-santhaya-namaha

Om-kaivasya sukathaya-namaha

Om-sachithananda vigrahaya-namaha

Om-jnanine-namaha

Om-dhayayuthaya-namaha - 80

Om-dandaya-namaha

Om-bahmad vesha vivarji thaya-namaha

Om-brahma thadaithya bayadaya-namaha

Om-kanttaya-namaha

Om-vibutheshwaraya-namaha

Om-ramarchitaya-namaha

Om-vadaye-namaha

Om-nagaraja yagnyoba veedhakaya-namaha

Om-stoolakanttaya-namaha

Om-svayam karthre-namaha - 90

Om-sama kosha priyaya-namaha

Om-parasmai-namaha

Om-stoolathundaya-namaha

Om-akranye-namaha

Om-deeraya-namaha

Om-vageesaya-namaha

Om-siddhithayakaya-namaha

Om-doorvapilvapriyaya-namaha

Om-avyakthamoorthayae-namaha

Om-athpuda moorthathi mathe-namaha - 100

Om-sailendradanu-namaha

Om-joth sanga kelanothsuka-namaha

Om-maanasaya-namaha

Om-svalavanya soodasara-namaha

Om-jitha manmade vikrahaya-namaha

Om-samastha jagatha daraya-namaha

Om- mayeenae -namaha

Om mooshikavahanaya-namaha – 108 (& more!)

Om-hrushtaya-namaha

Om-dushtaya-namaha

Om-prasannathmane-namaha

Om-shree sarva siddhi pradhayakaya-namaha

Note: After chanting above mantras, ring the bell and show the dhoop for Lord Ganesh. Then offer fruits or milk/ sweets to him. We can also light up ghee lamp or sesame oil lamp if required!

We can use most of the flowers or kumkum or holy ash or herbs like holi grass or bilva or holy rice (yellow rice – rice mixed with turmeric powder) for pooja / archana to perform with each names of Lord Ganesh. Keep image of Ganesh or idol, Sri Ganapathy chakram or photo, bell, dhoop, kumkum, chandan, fruits or milk/ sweets to offer him. Lemons or Holy Grass can also be used as maala or for archana. We can also light up ghee lamp or sesame oil lamp if required!

Then chant the following Ganapathy mantras one time each.

Ganesh Gayatri Mantra

Om Eka Thandhaya Vithmahe; Vakra Thundaya Dheemihi | Dhanno Dhandhi Prachotayad |

Om Vinayakaya Vithmahe; Vignarajaya Dheemihi | Dhanno Ganapathy Prachotayad |

[Below Ganapathy mantras are optional to chant!]

Shree Ganapathy Moola Mantra (simple version)

- Om Sreem Khreem Gleem Kloum Kam Ganapathiye Vara VaradevaSarva Janamme Vasamaanaya Swaha:
- Om Khlaam Kleem Kam Ganapathiye Vara Varadha mamah dhana dhaanya samruthim Dhehi Dhehi Swaha :
- Om Namo Vradha Pathaye Namo Ganapathaye' Namaha: Pramadha Pathaye' Namasthesthu Lambodharaya; Eka Thandhaya Vigna Vinasine, Siva Sudhaya Varadha Murthiye' Namo Namaha!
- Om sreem kam Soumyaya lakshmi ganapathiye' vara varadha sarva dhanamme vasamanaya swaha:
- Iym blum Om sreem hreem kleem kloum, Kam Ganapathiye' Vara Varadha Iym Blum Sarva Vidyam Dhehi Swaha:

Note: Finish the Ganapathy pooja prayers and do Varuna pooja next in a small vessel or bowl if possible.

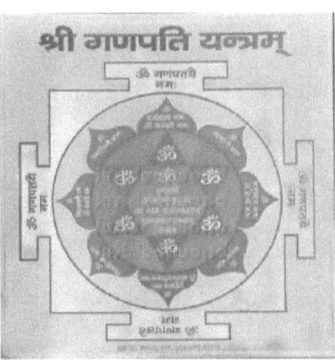

CHAPTER 4 – LORD VARUNA POOJA

You can keep another kalasam vessel for this purpose and decorate as shown for main kalasam. [or] Just put some flowers and a vessel of water with coconut and do the following chanting by putting flowers on it. This is very simple procedure. Once the pooja done, just sprinkle this water on you, the place where you do pooja or the whole house for holy cleansing.

Just say by keeping hand on the second small kalasam vessel or put yellow rice and flower on it; Then chant,

"Om imam mae varuna chruuthi-havam athyaacha hruthaya thvaama-vasyu raasakae asmin kalasae Sakala theertha-athipathim varunam aavaahayaami" [or] "Om Varuna Devatham Aavagayami" – 1 time as said above...*then, put flowers on the vessel and say.;*

Om Varunaaya Namaha : aasanam samar-payaami, pathayae : paathyam Smar-payaami, hasthayoa arkkiyam samar-payaami, aachama-niiyam Samar-payaami. Sthaapa-yaami, Snaanam aachama-neeyam samar-payaami, vasthram, aaparanaam. upaviitham akshatham samarpayaami, kanhtham samarpayaami, kungkumam samarpayaami.

Then again put flowers and chant;

Pushpam : pujayaami - Om varunaaya nama: prase-thasae nama: Svaruupinai nama: apaayam pathayae nama: paacha-hasthaaya nama: jalaathipathayae nama: makara vaahanaaya nama: varunaaya nama: .....

Note: After chanting above mantras, ring the bell and show the dhoop for Varuna devata. Then offer fruits or milk/ sweets to him. We can also light up ghee lamp or sesame oil lamp if required!

[Nhaanaa-vitha parimala pushpaani Samar-payaami…. Dhooba Dheepa akshathaan samar-payaami…… Dhupanartham aachama-niiyam samarppayaami…..(sprinkle some water) Om puur puvasva : Neivethanam samarpayami!....show fruits, milk or sweet etc.

Aachama-niiyam samarppayaami………(sprinkle some water again) Om puur puvasva :]

Then take some water from this vessel and sprinkle on you and your place fully to have the holy cleansing!

Then rest of the pooja starts!....

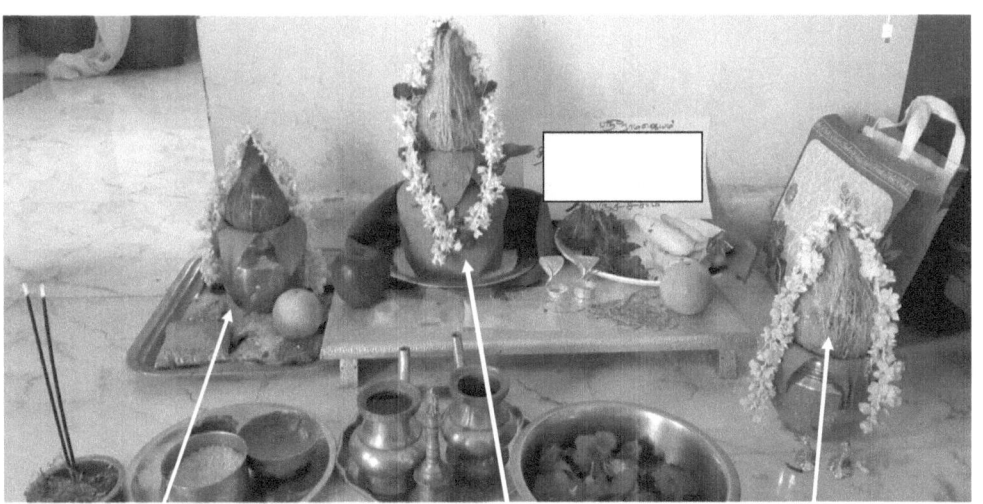

Navagraga Kalasam   Main Kalasam   Varuna Kalasam

Next Pooja is for Navagraga (9 planets). You can keep only 9 planets seeds or Navadanyam / one kalasam vessal as shown in the above picture. Or you can also do Navagraga pooja in the main kalasam vessel itself.

Start with "Om Navagraga Devatham Aavagayami" 1 time [or] "Surya, Chandra, Angaaraga, Budha, Guru, Chukra, Saneeswara devatham Aavagayami" 1 time. …..Put flowers (with yellow rice if possible) on kalasam vessel. …..Then do the below navagraga names chanting....put flowers…..

Add "Om" before and "Namaha" after each name [Ex: "Om Suryaya Namaha"]

Baanavae

Hamsaaya

Baaskaraaya

Surayaya

Suraaya

Thamoaharaaya

Rathinhae

Vishvathruthae'

Avyaapathrae'

Harayae   (10)

vaethamayaaya

vipavae

suththaamsavae

Supthaampavae

Chandraya

Apjanhaethra Samuthpavaya

Thaaraathipaaya

roahinee Saaya

Sumpumuurththi-kruthaalayaaya

Oashathiityaaya (20)

Oashathipathayae

Esvara tharaaya

Sudhanithayae

Sakalaahalaathanh tharaaya

Bowmaaya

BuumiSuthaaya

Puuthamaa nhyaaya

Samuthpava

Aaryaaya

Aknhikruthae   (30)

Roahithaangkaaya

Raktha vasthratharaaya

Susaye

Mangkalaaye'

Angkaarakaaya

Raktha maalainhae

Maayaavisaarathaaya

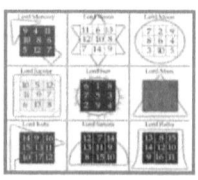

Buthaaya

ThaaraaSthaaya

Soumyaaya (40)

Roahineekarppa Sampuuthaa

Chanhthraathmajaaya

Soamavamparakaraaya

Churuthi vichaarathaaya

SathyaSanhthaaya

SathyaSinhthavae

Vithu Sthaaya

viputhaaya

Vipavae

Vaak kruthae (50)

Praahmanaa

Prahmanae

Thishanaaya

Supavaeshatharaaya -

Keeshpathayae

Kuravae

Inhthrapuroahithaaya

Jiivaaya

Nhirjara puujithaa

Piithaampara alangkruthaaya (60)

Prukavae

PaarkkavaSampuuthaaya

Nhichaachar kuravae

Kaviyae

Pruthyakaethaharaaya

Bruku Suthaaya

Varsha ruthe'

Theenaraajyathaaya

Sukraaya

SukraSvaruupaaye' (70)

Raajyathaaya

Layakruthaaya

Koanaaya

Sanhai Scharaaya

Manhthaaya

Chaayaa hiruthaya nhanhthanaaya

Maarthaandajaaya

Pangkavae

Paanhutha nhuupavaaya

Yamaanhujaaya (80)

Athipayakruthae

Nheelaaya

Suryavam Sajaaya

Nhirmaana thaehaaya

Raahavae

Svarpaanhavae

Aathithyachanhthrath vaeshinae

pujangkamaaya

Simhithae saaya

Kunavathe'   (90)

Raathripathipiitithaaya

Ahiraajae

Siro-hanhaaya

Vishatharaaya

Mahaakaayaaya

Mahaaputhaaya

Braahmanaa

Brahma Samputhaa

Ravikruthae

Raahu ruupathruthae (100)

Kaethavae

Kutu Svaruupaaya

Kaecha-raaya

Shukruthaa-layaaya

Prahma vithae

Prahma puthraaya

Kumaarakaaya

Praahmana prithaaya (108) ......then

Note: After chanting above mantras, ring the bell and show the dhoop for Navagraga Devatas. Then offer fruits or milk/ sweets to him. We can also light up ghee lamp or sesame oil lamp if required!

[if possible chant below to show all these dhoop, deep, fruits etc....]

[Nhaanaa-vitha parimala pushpaani Samar-payaami…. Dhooba Dheepa akshathaan samar-payaami…… Dhupanartham aachama-niiyam samarppayaami…..(sprinkle some water) Om puur puvasva :

Neivethanam samarpayami!....show fruits, milk or sweet etc.

Aachama-niiyam samarppayaami………(sprinkle some water again) Om puur puvasva :]

Then take some water from small bowl and sprinkle on kalasam vessel!

Then next…. Lakshmi pooja starts for main kalasam vessel!....

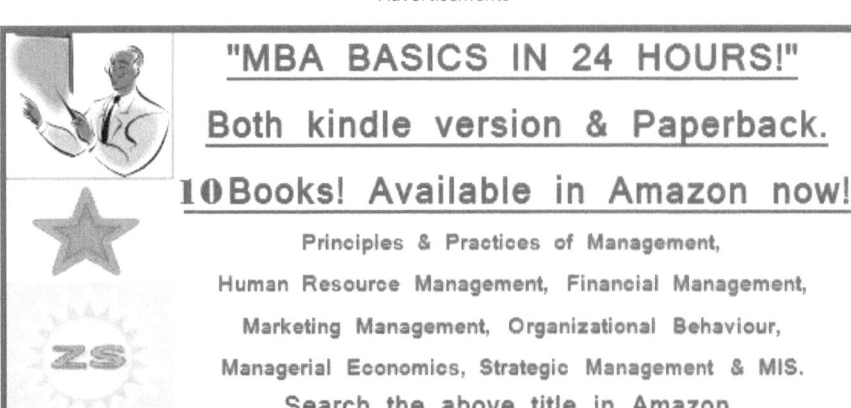
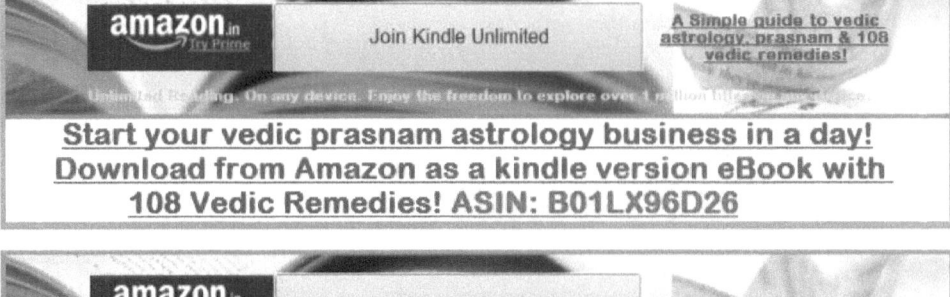
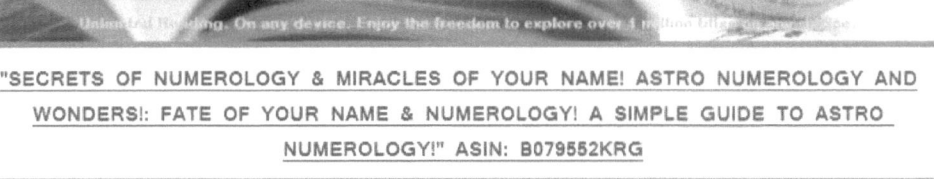

CHAPTER 6 – MAHAVISHNU/ MAHALAKSHMI POOJA

Put some flowers (with or without yellow rice/holy rice) and we are going to do all the angelic presence invocation at once. [It can be done individually also as per your wish before each deity/god/goddess pooja...we have already invocated Ganapathy, Varuna, Navagraga etc before... So you can continue the rest...]

Now we do all aavaganam (invocation together) each 1 time....

Om Mahavishu devatham Aavagayami

Om MahaLakshmi devatham Aavagayami

Om Hanuman devatham Aavagayami

Om Kula devatham Aavagayami [your family god if known]

Om Brahma devatham Aavagayami

Om Saraswathi devatham Aavagayami

Om Eeswara devatham Aavagayami

Om Gowri devatham Aavagayami

Om Varahi devatham Aavagayami

Om Pratyangra devatham Aavagayami

Om Sulini devatham Aavagayami

Om Maha Kaali devatham Aavagayami

Om Durga devatham Aavagayami

Om Lalitha devatham Aavagayami

Om Bala Thiripura Sundari devatham Aavagayami

Om Saptha Kanni devatham Aavagayami

Om Mirthyanja devatham Aavagayami

Om Nagaraja Swami devatham Aavagayami

Om Valli Devana sametha Subramanya devatham Aavagayami...........then,

Om Sarwa Devathaya Namaha : aasanam samar-payaami, Baathyam Smar-payaami, Arkkiyam samar-payaami, Aachama-niiyam Samar-payaami. Sthaapa-yaami, Snaanam aachama-neeyam samar-payaami, vasthram, aaparanaam. upaviitham akshatham samarpayaami, kanhtham samarpayaami, kungkumam samarpayaami. [put yellow rice or flowers on the main kalasam]

Then chant Vishnu Gayatri mantra: (keep putting flowers….)

OM NARAYANAYA VITHMAHE; VAASU DEVAYA DHEEMIHI,

DHANNO VISHNU PRACHOTHAYAD!

Om Achudaaya Namaha

Om Ananthaya Namaha

Om Govindaaya Namaha

Om Kesavaya Namaha

Om Narayanaaya Namaha

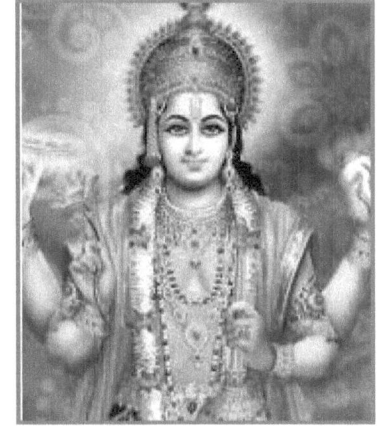

Om Maadhavaya Namaha

Om Govindaaya Namaha

Om Vishnuve Namaha

Om Madhusudhanaaya Namaha

Om Thiruvikramaaya Namaha

Om Vaamanaya Namaha

Om Sreedharaya Namaha

Om Rishikesaya Namaha

Om Padmanabaya Namaha

Om Dhamodharaaya Namaha

After these Mahavishnu names chanting; follow the next for Mahalakshmi…Offer flowers on Kalasam.

<u>This is Lakshmi Astothram….</u>

Om prakrityai Namaha .
Om vikrityai Namaha .
Om vidyaayai Namaha .
Om sarvabhuuta-hitapradaayai Namaha .
Om shraddhaayai Namaha .

Om vibhuutyai Namaha .
Om surabhyai Namaha .
Om paramaatmikaayai Namaha .
Om vaache Namaha .
Om padmaalayaayai Namaha .

Om padmaayai Namaha .
Om shuchaye Namaha .
Om svaahaayai Namaha .
Om svadhaayai Namaha .
Om sudhaayai Namaha .
Om dhanyaayai Namaha .
Om hiranmayyai Namaha .
Om laxmyai Namaha .
Om nityapushhtaayai Namaha .
Om vibhaavaryai Namaha .

Om adityai Namaha .
Om ditye Namaha .
Om diipaayai Namaha .
Om vasudhaayai Namaha .
Om vasudhaarinyai Namaha .
Om kamalaayai Namaha .
Om kaantaayai Namaha .
Om kaamaaxyai Namaha .
Om krodhasambhavaayai Namaha .
Om anugrahapradaayai Namaha .

Om buddhaye Namaha .
Om anaghaayai Namaha .
Om harivallabhaayai Namaha .
Om ashokaayai Namaha .
Om amritaayai Namaha .
Om diiptaayai Namaha .
Om lokashokavinaashinyai Namaha .

Om dharmanilayaayai Namaha .
Om karunaayai Namaha .
Om lokamaatre Namaha .

Om padmapriyaayai Namaha .
Om padmahastaayai Namaha .
Om padmaaxyai Namaha .
Om padmasundaryai Namaha .
Om padmodbhavaayai Namaha .
Om padmamukhyai Namaha .
Om padmanaabhapriyaayai Namaha .
Om ramaayai Namaha .
Om padmamaalaadharaayai Namaha .
Om devyai Namaha .

Om padminyai Namaha .
Om padmagandhinyai Namaha .
Om punyagandhaayai Namaha .
Om suprasannaayai Namaha .
Om prasaadaabhimukhyai Namaha .
Om prabhaayai Namaha .
Om diipaayai Namaha .
Om vasudhaayai Namaha .
Om vasudhaarinyai Namaha .
Om kamalaayai Namaha .

Om kaantaayai Namaha .
Om kaamaaxyai Namaha .
Om krodhasambhavaayai Namaha .
Om anugrahapradaayai Namaha .
Om buddhaye Namaha .
Om anaghaayai Namaha .
Om harivallabhaayai Namaha .
Om ashokaayai Namaha .
Om amritaayai Namaha .

Om diiptaayai Namaha .

Om lokashokavinaashinyai Namaha .
Om dharmanilayaayai Namaha .
Om karunaayai Namaha .
Om lokamaatre Namaha .
Om padmapriyaayai Namaha .
Om padmahastaayai Namaha .
Om padmaaxyai Namaha .
Om padmasundaryai Namaha .
Om padmodbhavaayai Namaha .
Om padmamukhyai Namaha .

Om padmanaabhapriyaayai Namaha .
Om ramaayai Namaha .
Om padmamaalaadharaayai Namaha .
Om devyai Namaha .
Om padminyai Namaha .
Om padmagandhinyai Namaha .
Om punyagandhaayai Namaha .
Om suprasannaayai Namaha .
Om prasaadaabhimukhyai Namaha .
Om prabhaayai Namaha .

Om diipaayai Namaha .
Om vasudhaayai Namaha .
Om vasudhaarinyai Namaha .
Om kamalaayai Namaha .
Om kaantaayai Namaha .
Om kaamaaxyai Namaha .
Om krodhasambhavaayai Namaha .
Om anugrahapradaayai Namaha .
Om buddhaye Namaha .
Om anaghaayai Namaha .

Om harivallabhaayai Namaha .
Om ashokaayai Namaha .
Om amritaayai Namaha .
Om diiptaayai Namaha .
Om lokashokavinaashinyai Namaha .
Om dharmanilayaayai Namaha .
Om karunaayai Namaha .
Om lokamaatre Namaha .
Om padmapriyaayai Namaha .
Om padmahastaayai Namaha .

Om padmaaxyai Namaha .
Om padmasundaryai Namaha .
Om padmodbhavaayai Namaha .
Om padmamukhyai Namaha .
Om padmanaabhapriyaayai Namaha .
Om ramaayai Namaha .
Om padmamaalaadharaayai Namaha .
Om devyai Namaha .
Om padminyai Namaha .
Om padmagandhinyai Namaha .

Om punyagandhaayai Namaha .
Om suprasannaayai Namaha .
Om prasaadaabhimukhyai Namaha .
Om prabhaayai Namaha .

Note: After chanting above mantras, ring the bell and show the dhoop for Mahavishnu/MahaLakshmi Devatas. Then offer fruits or milk/ sweets to him/her. We can also light up ghee lamp or sesame oil lamp if required!

[This is optional here...bcos, after finishing Hanuman pooja, it can be done]

[if possible chant below to show all these dhoop, deep, fruits etc....]

[Nhaanaa-vitha parimala pushpaani Samar-payaami.... Dhooba Dheepa akshathaan samar-payaami...... Dhupanartham aachama-niiyam samarppayaami.....(sprinkle some water) Om puur puvasva :

Neivethanam samarpayami!....show fruits, milk or sweet etc. Aachama-niiyam samarppayaami.........(sprinkle some water again) Om puur puvasva :]

Then take some water from small bowl and sprinkle on kalasam vessel!

Chant below Vishnu/lakshmi mantras 1 time.....

Vishnu Gayatri 1 time

Om Narayanaya Vithmahe | Vasudevaya Dheemihi | Dhanno Vishnu Prachotayad |

Mahavishnu Moola mantra

Om Sreem Kreem Kleem Narayanaya Swaha

Chant Lakshmi Gayatri 1 time

Om Mahadevi cha vithmahe | Vishnu pathni cha dheemihi | Dhanno Lakshmi Prachothayad|

MahaLakshmi Moola mantra

Om Sreem Kreem Kleem Maha Lakshmiye Swaha:

Then *next.... Hanuman Swami pooja starts* in main kalasam vessel!....

Start offering flowers in the main kalasam itself for chanting Hanuman ashtothram.....

CHAPTER 7 – HANUMAN / AANJANEYA POOJA

Chant Hanuman Gayatri &Moola mantra 1 time…..

Hanuman Gayatri Mantra

Om Aanjaneyaya Vithmahe; Maha Veeraya Dheemihi | Dhanno Hanuman Prachotayad |

Shree Hanuman Moola Mantra (simple version)

- **Om Hraam Hreem Hroom Hraim Hra Hum Bhat – Swaha:**

Shree Hanuman Ashtothra Namavali (108 names of Hanuman)

*Then chant the following **108** names of Hanuman!*

Om Angenayaya namah

Om Mahaveeraya namah

Om Hanumate namah

Om Marutatmajaya namah

Om Tatva-gnyana-pradaya namah

Om Sita-devi-mudhra-padraya kaya namah

Om Ashokavani-kaachetre namah

Om Sarva-maya-vibham-janaya namah

Om Sarva-banda-vimokthre namah

Om Raksho-vidhvamsa-karakaya namah - 10

Om Para-vidhya-pariharaya namah

Om Para-shourya-vinashanaya namah

Om Paramamtra-niraakarte namah

Om Parayantra-pradbedakaaya namah

Om Sarwagraha-vinaashine namah

Om Bhimasena-sahayakrute namah

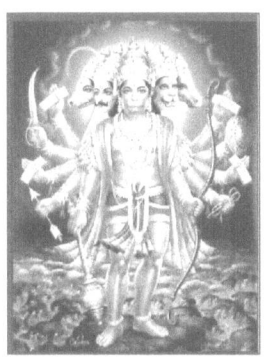

Om Sarwa-dukhaharaaya namah

Om Sarwa-lokachaarinye namah

Om Manojavaaya namah

Om Paarijaata drumulasdhaya namah - 20

Om Sarwa-mantra-swarupine namah

Om Sarwa-tantra-swarupine namah

Om Sarwa-yantratmakaaya namah

Om Kapeeshwaraaya namah

Om Mahakaayaaya namah

Om Sarwa-rogaharaaya namah

Om Prabhave namah

Om Balasiddhikaraaya namah

Om Sarwa-vidya-sampatpradaa-yakaaya namah

Om Kapisenaa-naayakaaya namah - 30

Om Bhavishya-chatu-rananaaya namah

Om Kumaara-bramhachaarine namah

Om Ratna-kundala-deeptamate namah

Om Sanchala-dwala-sannaddha-lambamaana shikhojwalaaya namah

Om Gandharwa-vidya-tatwagnyaya namah

Om Mahabala-paraakramaaya namah

Om Kaaraa-gruha-vimoktre namah

Om Shrumkhalaa-bandhamochakaaya namah

Om Saagarottarakaaya namah

Om Pragnyaya namah - 40

Om Raama-dhutaaya namah

Om Prataapavate namah

Om Vaanaraaya namah

Om Kesaree-sutaaya namah

Om Seetaa-shoka-nivaaranaaya namah

Om Amjanaa-garbha-sambhutaaya namah

Om Baalaarka-sadrushaananaaya namah

Om Vibhishana-priyakaraaya namah

Om Dhashagreva-kulaamtakaaya namah

Om Lakshana-pranadaataaya namah - 50

Om Vajra-kaayaaya namah

Om Mahadyutaye namah

Om Chinrajeevine namah

Om Raamabhaktaya namah

Om Daitya-kaarya-vighatakaaya namah

Om Akshahamtre namah

Om Kaancha-naabhaya namah

Om Pancha-vaktraya namah

Om Maha-tapaaya namah

Om Lamkhinee-bhamjanaaya namah - 60

Om Srimate namah

Om Simhaka-pranabhamjanaaya namah

Om Gandha-maadana-sailasdhaya namah

Om Lankaa-puravidaahakaaya namah

Om Sugriva-sachi-vaaya namah

Om Ddhiraaya namah

Om Shuraya namah

Om Daityakulamtakaaya namah

Om Suraarchitaaya namah

Om Mahatejaaya namah - 70

Om Raama-chudaa-manipradaaya namah

Om Kaama-rupaaya namah

Om Pingalakshaya namah

Om Vaardhi-mainaaka-pujitaaya namah

Om Kabali-kruta-martamda-mamdalaaya namah

Om Vijitem-driyaaya namah

Om Raama-sugriva-samdhaatre namah

Om Maha-raavana-mardhanaaya namah

Om Spatikaabhaya namah

Om Vaagadhishaya namah - 80

Om Navavya-kruti-panditaaya namah

Om Chatur-bahave namah

Om Deena-bandhave namah

Om Mahatmaya namah

Om Bhaktha-vastalaaya namah

Om Sanjeeva-vanaanna-graharthe namah

Om Shuchaye namah

Om Vaagmine namah

Om Drudavrataaya namah

Om Kaalaneme-pramadha-naaya namah - 90

Om Hari-markata-markataaya namah

Om Damtaaya namah

Om Shantaaya namah

Om Prasanaatmane namah

Om Shatakanta-madaapahrute namah

Om Yogine namah

Om Raamakadhalolaaya namah

Om Seetaanveshana-panditaaya namah

Om Vajra-damstraya namah

Om Vajranakhaya namah - 100

Om Rudhra-veerya-samudbavaaya namah

Om Indhra-jitpra-hitaa-mogha bramhastra nivaarakaaya namah

Om Paardha-dhwajaagra-samvaasine namah

Om Shara-panjara-bhedhakaaya namah

Om Dashabaahave namah

Om Lokapujyayaa namah

Om Jaamba-vatpri-tiva-rdhanaaya namah

Om Seetaa-sameta sreeraamapaada sevaa Duramdharaaya namah -108

Note: After chanting above mantras, ring the bell and show the dhoop for Lord Hanuman. Then offer fruits or milk/ sweets to him. We can also light up ghee lamp or sesame oil lamp if required!

[if possible chant below to show all these dhoop, deep, fruits etc....]

[Nhaanaa-vitha parimala pushpaani Samar-payaami…. Dhooba Dheepa akshathaan samar-payaami…… Dhupanartham aachama-niiyam samarppayaami…..(sprinkle some water) Om puur puvasva : Neivethanam samarpayami!....show fruits, milk or sweet etc.

Aachama-niiyam samarppayaami………(sprinkle some water again) Om puur puvasva :]

Then take some water from small bowl and sprinkle on kalasam vessel!

Then next…. Varahi Devi pooja starts in main kalasam vessel!....

Start offering flowers in the main kalasam itself for chanting Varahi ashtothram/ other mantras…..

CHAPTER 8 – VARAHI DEVI POOJA

Chant Varahi Devi Gayatri & Moola mantra 1 time.....

Varahi Gayatri Mantra

Om Varaha Mukyai Vithmahe; Dhanda-nathaya Dheemihi | Dhanno Harigiri Prachotayad |

Shree Varahi Moola Mantras

Aam - hreem – krom – yaehi –parameshwari – swaha:

Shree Varahi Veeya Namavali (12 names of varahi)

Then chant the following 12 names of Varahi...offer flowers!

- ❖ Om Panchami -namaha
- ❖ Om Dandanatha -namaha
- ❖ Om Sangketha -namaha
- ❖ Om Sameshwari -namaha
- ❖ Om Samaya Sangketha -namaha
- ❖ Om Varahi -namaha
- ❖ Om Bothrini -namaha
- ❖ Om Sivaya -namaha
- ❖ Om Vaarthali -namaha
- ❖ Om Maha Sena -namaha
- ❖ Om Anja chakreshwari -namaha
- ❖ Om Arigni -namaha

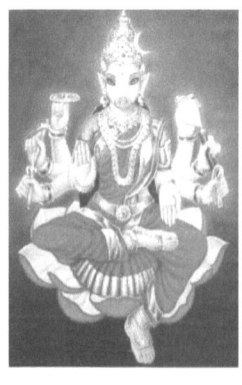

Shree Varahi Ashtothra Sadha Namavali

Then chant the following 108 names of Varahi! This includes some beeja mantras which gives powerful siddhis which can be realised by varahi devi blessings only., also very powerful remedy for many bad planetary positions!

Om -iym-kloum-varahyai-namaha

Om -iym-kloum-panjami siddhi devyai-namaha

Om -iym-kloum-vasvyai-namaha

Om -iym-kloum-vaidehyai-namaha

Om -iym-kloum-vasudhayai-namaha

Om -iym-kloum- Vishnu vallabhayai-namaha

Om -iym-kloum-balayai-namaha

Om -iym-kloum-vasundharayai-namaha

Om -iym-kloum-vamayai-namaha

Om -iym-kloum-darminyai-namaha - 10

Om -iym-kloum-adisayakarya siddhitayai-namaha

Om -iym-kloum-bagavathyai-namaha

Om -iym-kloum-shree purarakshinyai-namaha

Om -iym-kloum-vanapriyayai-namaha

Om -iym-kloum-kamyayai-namaha

Om -iym-kloum-kanjanyai-namaha

Om -iym-kloum-kabalinyai-namaha

Om -iym-kloum-darayai-namaha

Om -iym-kloum-lakshmyai-namaha

Om -iym-kloum-sakthyai-namaha - 20

Om -iym-kloum-sandyai-namaha

Om -iym-kloum-beemayai-namaha

Om -iym-kloum-abayayai-namaha

Om -iym-kloum-vaarthalyai-namaha

Om -iym-kloum-vakvilasinyai-namaha

Om -iym-kloum-nithya vaihbhavayai-namaha

Om -iym-kloum-nithya sandhoshinyai-namaha

Om -iym-kloum-manimaguda bushanayai-namaha

Om -iym-kloum-manimandaba vasinyai-namaha

Om -iym-kloum-rakthamal yam baratharayai-namaha -30

Om -iym-kloum- kabala priyadandinyai-namaha

Om -iym-kloum-asvaroodayai-namaha

Om -iym-kloum-dandanayakyai-namaha

Om -iym-kloum-kirichakra radharoodayai-namaha

Om -iym-kloum-utharayai-namaha

Om -iym-kloum-varahamukayai-namaha

Om -iym-kloum-bairavayai-namaha

Om -iym-kloum-kurkurayai-namaha

Om -iym-kloum-varunyai-namaha

Om -iym-kloum-brummarandha rakayai-namaha -40

Om -iym-kloum-svargayai-namaha

Om -iym-kloum-padalakayai-namaha

Om -iym-kloum-boomikayai-namaha

Om -iym-kloum-sriyai-namaha

Om -iym-kloum-asidharinyai-namaha

Om -iym-kloum-karkarayai-namaha

Om -iym-kloum-manovasayai-namaha

Om -iym-kloum-andhe andhinyai-namaha

Om -iym-kloum-chaturanga balodkatayai-namaha

Om -iym-kloum-sathyayai-namaha -50

Om -iym-kloum-kshetragnyayai-namaha

Om -iym-kloum-mangalayai-namaha

Om -iym-kloum-mruthyai-namaha

Om -iym-kloum-mrutyunjayayai-namaha

Om -iym-kloum-mahishagnyai-namaha

Om -iym-kloum-simharoodayai-namaha

Om -iym-kloum-mahisharoodayai-namaha

Om -iym-kloum-vyakra roodayai-namaha

Om -iym-kloum-asvaroodayai-namaha

Om -iym-kloum-runderundinyai-namaha - 60

Om -iym-kloum-danyapradayai-namaha

Om -iym-kloum-darapradayai-namaha

Om -iym-kloum-papanasinyai-namaha

Om -iym-kloum-doshanasinyai-namaha

Om -iym-kloum-ripunasinyai-namaha

Om -iym-kloum-kshmaroopinyai-namaha

Om -iym-kloum-siddhidayinyai-namaha

Om -iym-kloum-roudryai-namaha

Om -iym-kloum-sarvagnyayai-namaha

Om -iym-kloum-vyadinasinyai-namaha - 70

Om -iym-kloum-abaya varadhayai-namaha

Om -iym-kloum-jambejambinyai-namaha

Om -iym-kloum-uthandinyai-namaha

Om -iym-kloum-dandanayikayai-namaha

Om -iym-kloum-dukkanasinyai-namaha

Om -iym-kloum-daaridraya nasinyai-namaha

Om -iym-kloum-hiranya kavasayai-namaha

Om -iym-kloum-vyasavaa ayyyikayai-namaha

Om -iym-kloum-arishta thamanyai-namaha

Om -iym-kloum-samundayai-namaha - 80

Om -iym-kloum-kandhinyai-namaha

Om -iym-kloum-gorakshakayai-namaha

Om -iym-kloum-boomithanesh waryai-namaha

Om -iym-kloum-mohemohinyai-namaha

Om -iym-kloum-bahuroopayai-namaha

Om -iym-kloum-svapnavarahyai-namaha

Om -iym-kloum-mahavarahyai-namaha

Om -iym-kloum-aashata panjami boojana priyayai-namaha

Om -iym-kloum-madhu varahyai-namaha

Om -iym-kloum-manthrini varahyai-namaha -90

Om -iym-kloum-bakthavarahyai-namaha

Om -iym-kloum-panjamyai-namaha

Om -iym-kloum-panjika peedavasinyai-namaha

Om -iym-kloum-sanjethayai-namaha

Om -iym-kloum-samayeshwaryai-namaha

Om -iym-kloum-stambes thambinyai-namaha

Om -iym-kloum-vanavasinyai-namaha

Om -iym-kloum-kruparupinyai-namaha

Om -iym-kloum-dayarupinyai-namaha

Om -iym-kloum-sakalavigna vinasinyai-namaha -100

Om -iym-kloum-bothrinyai-namaha

Om -iym-kloum-sarvadushta jihvamugavark stambinyai-namaha

Om -iym-kloum-anungrahatayai-namaha

Om -iym-kloum-anima siddhitayai-namaha

Om -iym-kloum-shree bruhat varahyai-namaha

Om -iym-kloum-aagnya chakreshwaryai-namaha

Om -iym-kloum-visvavijayayai-namaha

Om -iym-kloum-shree bhuvaneshwari priya maha varahyai-namaha - 108

Note:

- After chanting above mantras, ring the bell and show the dhoop for Goddess Kaali Varahi. Then offer fruits or milk/ sweets to her. We can also light up ghee lamp or sesame oil lamp if required! [Or this can be done after finishing other Devi poojas & Mirthyanja pooja also]

Then next…. Gowri Devi pooja starts in main kalasam vessel!….

Start offering flowers in the main kalasam itself for chanting Gowri ashtothram/ other mantras…..

CHAPTER 9 – GOWRI DEVI POOJA

Chant Gowri Devi Gayatri & Moola mantra 1 time.....

Gowri Gayatri Mantra

Om Mahadevicha Vithmahe; Eeshwara Pathicha Dheemihi | Dhanno Parvathi Prachotayad |

Shree Gowri Moola Mantra

Om Sreem; Kreem, Gleem Maha Gowriye' Namaha:

Then Offer flowers/ Akshadha (yellow rice) in main kalasam and chant the Gowri devi 108 names. **(Gowri Asthothram 108 names)**

Om Shree gauryai Namaha
Om Ganesha jananyai Namaha
Om Guhambi kayai Namaha
Om Jaga nnetryai Namaha
Om Giritanu bhavayai Namaha
Om Veera bhadra prasuve Namaha
Om Vishva vyapinyai Namaha
Om Vishva rupinyai Namaha
Om Ashta murtyat mekayai Namaha
Om Ashta daridrya shamanyai Namaha   10
Om Shivayai Namaha
Om Shambha vayai Namaha
Om Shan karyai Namaha
Om Balaayai Namaha
Om Bhavanyai Namaha
Om Haima vatyai Namaha
Om Parvatyai Namaha
Om Papa nasinyai Namaha
Om Narayanam shajaayai Namaha
Om Nityayai Namaha   20
Om Nirma laayai Namaha
Om Ambi kayai Namaha

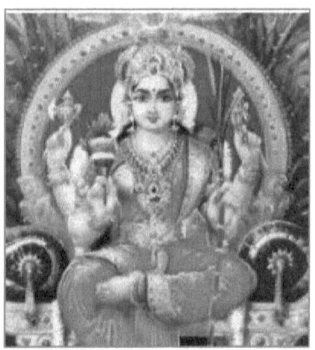

Om Hemadri jaayai Namaha
Om Vedanta lakshanayai Namaha
Om Karma bramha mayai Namaha
Om Ganga dhara kutumbinyai Namaha
Om Mrudanyai Namaha
Om Muni samsevyayai Namaha
Om Maninyai Namaha
Om Menakat majaayai Namaha   30
Om Kumaryai Namaha
Om Kanyakayai Namaha
Om Durgayai Namaha
Om Kalidosha vighatinyai Namaha
Om Katya yanyai Namaha
Om Bhadra daenyai Namaha
Om Mangalya daenyai Namaha
Om Sarva mangalayai Namaha
Om Manju bhashinyai Namaha
Om Mahe shvaryai Namaha   40
Om Maha mayayai Namaha
Om Mantra radhyayai Namaha
Om Maha balayai Namaha
Om Satyai Namaha
Om Sarva mayai Namaha
Om Soubhagya dayai Namaha
Om Kama kala nayai Namaha
Om Kamkshi tardha pradayai Namaha
Om Chandrarka yuta tatamkayai Namaha
Om Chidambara shareerinyai Namaha 50
Om Sree chakra vasinyai Namaha
Om Devyai Namaha
Om Kameshva rapatyai Namaha
Om Kamalayai Namaha
Om Murari priyardhamgyai Namaha
Om Putra poutra varapradayai Namaha
Om Punyayai Namaha

Om Krupa prurnayai Namaha
Om Kalyanyai Namaha
Om Anchit yayai Namaha   60
Om Tripurayai Namaha
Om Trigunam bikayai Namaha
Om Purushardha pradayai Namaha
Om Satya dharma ratayai Namaha
Om Sarva sakshinyai Namaha
Om Shashamka rupinyai Namaha
Om Sarasvatyai Namaha
Om Virajayai Namaha
Om Svahayai Namaha
Om Svadhayai Namaha   70
Om Pratyamgi rambikayai Namaha
Om Aaryayai Namaha
Om Dakshaenyai Namaha
Om Deekshayai Namaha
Om Sarvottamotta mayai Namaha
Om Shivabhinama deyayai Namaha
Om Sreevidyayai Namaha
Om Pranavardha svarupinyai Namaha
Om Hrinkaryai Namaha
Om Naada rupayai Namaha   80
Om Sundaryai Namaha
Om Shodashakshara devatayai Namaha
Om Mahagouryai Namaha
Om Shyamalayai Namaha
Om Chandyai Namaha
Om Bhaga malinyai Namaha
Om Bhagalayai Namaha
Om Matrukayai Namaha
Om Shulinyai Namaha
Om Amalayai Namaha   90
Om Annapurnayai Namaha
Om Akhilagama samstut yayai Namaha

Om Ambayai Namaha
Om Bhanukoti sandyatayai Namaha
Om Parayai Namaha
Om Seetamshu kruta shekha rayai Namaha
Om Sarvakala sumangalyai Namaha
Om Soma shekharyai Namaha
Om Amara samsev yayai Namaha
Om Amrutai shvaryai Namaha   100
Om Sukha sachi chudara sayai Namaha
Om Balyaradita bhutidayai Namaha
Om Hiranyayai Namaha
Om Sukshmayai Namaha
Om Haridra kumkuma radhyayai Namaha
Om Sarvabhoga pradayai Namaha
Om Markandeya varapradayai Namaha

Om Sree nityagouree devatayai Namaha   108

Note:

- After chanting above mantras, ring the bell and show the dhoop for Goddess Gowri (Parvathi). Then offer fruits or milk/ sweets to her. We can also light up ghee lamp or sesame oil lamp if required! [Or this can be done after finishing other Devi poojas & Mirthyanja pooja also]

Then next…. Durga Devi pooja starts in main kalasam vessel!….

Start offering flowers in the main kalasam itself for chanting Durga ashtothram/ other mantras…..

CHAPTER 10 – DURGA DEVI POOJA

Chant Durga Devi Gayatri & Moola mantra 1 time.....

Durga Gayatri Mantra

Om Gaatyaya Naaya Vithmahe; Kanya Kumaari Dheemihi | Dhanno Durge' Prachotayad |

Shree Durga Moola Mantra

Om Sreem; Kreem, Gleem Maha Durga Devi-yai Namaha:

Then Offer flowers/ Akshadha (yellow rice) in main kalasam and chant the Durga devi 108 names (Ashtothram).

Durga Devi Ashtothram (108 names)

Om Drugayai Namaha

Om Shivayai Namaha

Om Mahalakshmyai Namaha

Om Mahagouryai Namaha

Om Chandikaye Namaha

Om Sarvagynayai Namaha

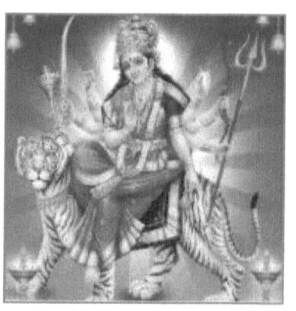

Om Sarvalokeshayai Namaha

Om Sarva karmaphalapradayai Namaha

Om Sarva teerdhamayai Namaha

Om Punyayai Namaha

Om Devayonaye Namaha

Om Ayonijaayai Namaha

Om Bhyai Namaha

Om Nirgunayai Namaha

Om Aadharashaktyai Namaha   (15)

Om Aaneeshvaryai Namaha

Om Nirgunayai Namaha

Om Niramhamkarayai Namaha

Om Sarvagarvavimardhinyai Namaha

Om Sarvalokapriyayai Namaha

Om Vaanyai Namaha

Om Sarvavidyadhidevataayai Namaha

Om Parvatyai Namaha

Om Devamatre Namaha

Om Vaneeshayai Namaha

Om Vindyavasinyai Namaha

Om Tejovatyai Namaha

Om Mahamatre Namaha

Om Kotisuryasamaprabhayai Namaha

Om Devatayai Namaha   (30)

Om Vahnirupayai Namaha

Om Satejase Namaha

Om Varnarupinyai Namaha

Om Gunashayayai Namaha

Om Gunamadhyayai Namaha

Om Gunatrayavivarjitayai Namaha

Om Karmagynanapradayai Namaha

Om Kantayai Namaha

Om Sarvasamharakarinyai Namaha

Om Dharmagynanayai Namaha

Om Dharmanistayai Namaha

Om Sarvakarmavivardhitayai Namaha

Om Kamakshmai Namaha

Om Kamasamhartyai Namaha

Om Kamakrodhavivarjitayai Namaha   (45)

Om Shankaryai Namaha

Om Shambhavyai Namaha

Om Shantayai Namaha

Om Chandrasuryagnilochanayai Namaha

Om Sujayayai Namaha

Om Jayabhumishtayai Namaha

Om Jaahnavyai Namaha

Om Janapujitayai Namaha

Om Shastrasyai Namaha

Om Shastramayyai Namaha

Om Nityayai Namaha

Om Shubhayai Namaha

Om Chandhrardhamastakayai Namaha

Om Bharatyai Namaha

Om Bramaryai Namaha   (60)

Om Kalpayai Namaha

Om Karalyai Namaha

Om Krushanapingalayai Namaha

Om Bramhai Namaha

Om Narayanyai Namaha

Om Roudryai Namaha

Om Chandramrutaparisrutayai Namaha

Om Jyeshtayai Namaha

Om Indirayai Namaha

Om Mahamayayai Namaha

Om Jagatgrushtyadhikarinyai Namaha

Om Bramhandakotisam sdhanayai Namaha

Om Kaminyai Namaha

Om Kamalaalayayai Namaha

Om katyayanyai Namaha   (75)

Om Kalaateetayai Namaha

Om Kalasamharakarinyai Namaha

Om Yoganishtayai Namaha

Om Yogigamyayai Namaha

Om Yogidyeyayai Namaha

Om Tapasvinyai Namaha

Om Gynanapupayai Namaha

Om Nirakarayai Namaha

Om Bhaktabhishtaphalapradayai Namaha

Om Bhutatmekayai Namaha

Om Bhutamatre Namaha

Om Bhuteshyai Namaha

Om Bhutadarinyai Namaha

Om Svadhayai Namaha

Om Nareemadhyagatayai Namaha   (90)

Om Shadadharadivardhinyai Namaha

Om Mohitamshubhadayai Namaha

Om Shubhrayai Namaha

Om Sukshmayai Namaha

Om Matrayai Namaha

Om Niralasayai Namaha

Om Nimnagayai Namaha

Om Neelasamkashayai Namaha

Om Nityanandayai Namaha

Om Harayai Namaha

Om Paraayai Namaha

Om Sarvagynanapradayai Namaha

Om Anamtayai Namaha

Om Satyayai Namaha

Om Durlabharupinyai Namaha

Om Sarasvatyai Namaha

Om Sarvagatayai Namaha

Om Sarvabheeshtapradainyai Namaha   (108)

Note:

- After chanting above mantras, ring the bell and show the dhoop for Goddess Durga. Then offer fruits or milk/ sweets to her. We can also light up ghee lamp or sesame oil lamp if required! [Or this can be done after finishing other Devi poojas & Mirthyanja pooja also]

Then next....Saraswathi Devi pooja starts in main kalasam vessel!....

Start offering flowers in the main kalasam itself for chanting Saraswathi ashtothram/ other mantras.

CHAPTER 11 – SARASWATHI DEVI POOJA

Chant Saraswathi Devi Gayatri & Moola mantra 1 time…..

Saraswathi Gayatri Mantra

Om Vaak Devi Cha Vithmahe; Virinji Pathni Cha Dheemihi | Dhanno Vaani Prachotayad |

Saraswathi Moola Mantra

Om Sreem; Kreem, Gleem Maha Saraswathi-yai Namaha:

Then Offer flowers/ Akshadha (yellow rice) in main kalasam and chant the Saraswathi devi 108 names (Ashtothram).

Saraswathi Devi Ashtothram (108 names)

Om sarasvatyai Namaha
Om mahabhadrayai Namaha
Om mahamayayai Namaha
Om varapradayai Namaha
Om padmanilayayai Namaha
Om padma kṣraiya Namaha
Om padmavaktrayai Namaha
Om śivanujayai Namaha
Om pusta kadhrate Namaha
Om ṅñana samudrayai Namaha   10
Om ramayai Namaha
Om parayai Namaha
Om kamara rūpayai Namaha
Om maha vidyayai Namaha
Om mahapata kanaśinyai Namaha
Om mahaśrayayai Namaha
Om malinyai Namaha
Om mahabhogayai Namaha
Om mahabhujayai Namaha
Om mahabhagyayai Namaha   20

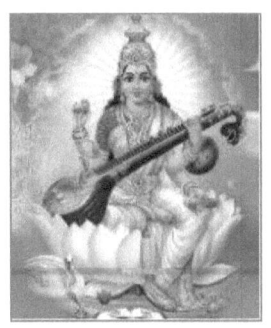

Om mahotsahayai Namaha
Om divyaṅgayai Namaha
Om suravanditayai Namaha
Om mahakaḷyai Namaha
Om mahapaśayai Namaha
Om mahakarayai Namaha
Om mahaṅkuśayai Namaha
Om sītayai Namaha
Om vimalayai Namaha
Om viśvayai Namaha   30
Om vidyunmalayai Namaha
Om vaiṣṇavyai Namaha
Om candrikayyai Namaha
Om candravadanayai Namaha
Om candra lekhavibhūṣitayai Namaha
Om savitryai Namaha
Om surasayai Namaha
Om devyai Namaha
Om divyalaṅkara bhūṣitayai Namaha
Om vagdevyai Namaha   40
Om vasudhayyai Namaha
Om tīvrayai Namaha
Om mahabhadrayai Namaha
Om maha balayai Namaha
Om bhogadayai Namaha
Om bharatyai Namaha
Om bhamayai Namaha
Om govindayai Namaha
Om gOmatyai Namaha
Om śivayai Namaha
Om jaṭilayai Namaha
Om vindhyavasayai Namaha
Om vindhyacala virajitayai Namaha
Om caṇḍi kayai Namaha
Om vaiṣṇavyai Namaha

Om brahmyai Namaha
Om brahmaṅña naikasadhanayai Namaha
Om saudamanyai Namaha
Om sudha mūrtyai Namaha
Om subhadrayai Namaha 60
Om sura pūjitayai Namaha
Om suvasinyai Namaha
Om sunasayai Namaha
Om vinidrayai Namaha
Om padmalocanayai Namaha
Om vidya rūpayai Namaha
Om viśalakṣyai Namaha
Om brahmajayayai Namaha
Om maha phalayai Namaha
Om trayīmūrtyai Namaha 70
Om trikalaṅñaye Namaha
Om triguṇayai Namaha
Om śastra rūpiṇyai Namaha
Om śumbha surapramadinyai Namaha
Om śubhadayai Namaha
Om sarvatmikayai Namaha
Om rakta bījanihantryai Namaha
Om camuṇḍayai Namaha
Om ambikayai Namaha
Om manṇakaya praharaṇayai Namaha 80
Om dhūmralocanamardanayai Namaha
Om sarvade vastutayai Namaha
Om saumyayai Namaha
Om sura sura namaskratayai Namaha
Om kaḷa ratryai Namaha
Om kaladharayai Namaha
Om rūpasaubhagyadayinyai Namaha
Om vagdevyai Namaha
Om vararohayai Namaha
Om varahyai Namaha 90

Om vari jasanayai Namaha
Om citrambarayai Namaha
Om citra gandha yai Namaha
Om citra malya vibhūṣitayai Namaha
Om kantayai Namaha
Om kamapradayai Namaha
Om vandyayai Namaha
Om vidyadhara supūjitayai Namaha
Om śvetananayai Namaha
Om nīlabhujayai Namaha   100
Om caturvarga phalapradayai Namaha
Om caturanana samrajyai Namaha
Om rakta madhyayai Namaha
Om nirañjanayai Namaha
Om haṃsasanayai Namaha
Om nīlañjaṅghayai Namaha
Om Sri pradayai Namaha
Om brahmaviṣṇu śivatmikayai Namaha 108

Note:

- After chanting above mantras, ring the bell and show the dhoop for Goddess Saraswathi. Then offer fruits or milk/ sweets to her. We can also light up ghee lamp or sesame oil lamp if required! [Or this can be done after finishing other Devi poojas & Mirthyanja pooja also]

Then next…. Lalitha Devi pooja starts in main kalasam vessel!….

Start offering flowers in the main kalasam itself for chanting Lalitha ashtothram/ other mantras…..[mantras are bit difficult for lalitha… you can manage]…

CHAPTER 12 – LALITHA DEVI POOJA

Chant Lalitha Devi Gayatri & Moola mantra 1 time…..

Lalitha Gayatri Mantra

Om Lalitha Devi-cha Vithmahe; Kaameshwar-ya Dheemihi | Dhanno Devi Prachotayad |

Shree Lalitha Moola Mantra

Om Sreem; Kreem, Gleem Lalitha Devi-yai Namaha:

Then Offer flowers/ Akshadha (yellow rice) in main kalasam and chant the Lalitha devi 108 names (Ashtothram).

Lalitha Devi Ashtothram (108 names)

Om Rajataachala-shringaagra madhyasthaayai namo Namaha

Om Himaachalamahaavansha paavanaayai namo Namaha

Om   Shankarardhangasaundarya shariiraayai namo Namaha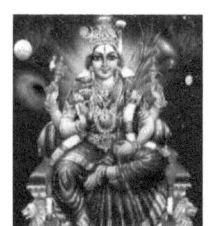

Om Lasanmarakatasvachchha vigrahaayai namo Namaha

Om Mahaatishayasaundarya laavanyaayai namo Namaha

Om Shashaankashekharapraana vallabhaayai namo Namaha

Om Sadaapanchadashaatmaikya svaruupaayai namo Namaha

Om Vajramaanikyakataka kiriitaayai namo Namaha

Om Kasturiitilakollasa nitilaayai namo Namaha

Om Bhasmarekhaankitalasan mastakaayai namo Namaha   10

Om Vikachaambhoruhadala lochanaayai namo Namaha

Om Sharaccampeyapushpaabha naasikaayai namo Namaha

Om Lasatkaanchanataatanka yugalaayai namo Namaha

Om Manidarpanasankaasha kapolaayai namo Namaha

Om Taambulapuritasmera vadanaayai namo Namaha

Om Supakvadaadimiibiija radanaayai namo Namaha

Om Kambupugasamachchaaya kandharaayai namo Namaha

Om Sthuulamuktaaphalodaara suhaaraayai namo Namaha

Om Giriishabaddhamaangalya mangalaayai namo Namaha

Om Padmapaashaankushalasat karaabjaayai namo Namaha   20

Om Padmakairavamandaara sumaalinyai namo Namaha

Om Suvarnakumbhayugmaabha sukuchaayai namo Namaha

Om Ramaniiyachaturbaahu sanyuktaayai namo Namaha

Om Kanakaangadakeyuura bhuushitaayai namo Namaha

Om Brihatsauvarnasaundarya vasanaayai namo Namaha

Om Brihannitambavilasajja ghanaayai namo Namaha

Om Saubhaagyajaatashringaara madhyamaayai namo Namaha

Om Divyabhuushanasandoha ranjitaayai namo Namaha

Om Paarijatagunaadhikya padaabjaayai namo Namaha

Om Supadmaraagasankaasha charanaayai namo Namaha   30

Om Kaamakotimahaapadma piithasthaayai namo Namaha

Om Shriikamthanetrakumuda chandrikaayai namo Namaha

Om Sanchaaramararamaavaanii viijitaayai namo Namaha

Om Bhaktarakshanadaakshinya kataakshaayai namo Namaha

Om Bhuuteshaalinganodbhuuta pulakaangyai namo Namaha

Om Anangajanakaapaanga viikshanaayai namo Namaha

Om Brahmopendrashiroratna ranjitaayai namo Namaha

Om Shachiimukhyaamaravadhuu sevitaayai namo Namaha

Om Liilaakalpitabrahmaanda mandalaayai namo Namaha

Om Amritaadimahaashakti sanvritaayai namo Namaha   40

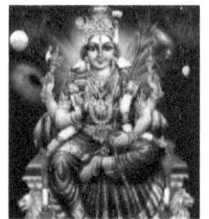

Om Ekaatapatrasaamraajya daayikaayai namo Namaha

Om Sanakaadisamaaraadhya paadukaayai namo Namaha

Om Devarshibhisstuuyamaana vaibhavaayai namo Namaha

Om Kalashodbhavadurvaasah puujitaayai namo Namaha

Om Mattebhavaktrashadvaktra vatsalaayai namo Namaha

Om Chakraraajamahaayantra madhya vartinyai namo Namaha

Om Chidagnikundasambhuuta sudehaayai namo Namaha

Om Shashaankakhandasanyukta makutaayai namo Namaha

Om Mattahansavadhuumanda gamanaayai namo Namaha

Om Vandaarujanasandoha vanditaayai namo Namaha   50

Om Antarmukhajanaananda phaladaayai namo Namaha

Om Pativrataanganaabhiishta phaladaayai namo Namaha

Om Avyaajakarunaapura puritaayai namo Namaha

Om Nitaantasaccidaananda sanyuktaayai namo Namaha

Om Sahasrasuryasanyukta prakaashaayai namo Namaha

Om Ratnachintaamanigriha madhyasthaayai namo Namaha

Om Haanivriddhigunaadhikya rahitaayai namo Namaha

Om Mahaapadmaataviimadhya nivaasaayai namo Namaha

Om Jagratsvapnasushuptiinaan saakshibhuutyai namo Namaha

Om Mahaapaapaughapaapaanaan vinaashinyai namo Namaha   60

Om Dushtabhiitimahaabhiiti bhanjanaayai namo Namaha

Om Samastadevadanujap rerakaayai namo Namaha

Om Samastahridayaambhuuja nilayaayai namo Namaha

Om Anaahatamahaapadmama ndiraayai namo Namaha

Om Sahasraarasarojaata vaasitaayai namo Namaha

Om Punaraavrittirahita purasthaayai namo Namaha

Om Vaanigaayatrisaavitri sannutaayai namo Namaha

Om Ramaabhuumisutaaraadhya padaabjaayai namo Namaha

Om Lopaamudraarchitashrima ccaranaayai namo Namaha

Om Sahasraratisaundarya shariraayai namo Namaha   70

Om Bhaavanaamaatrasantushta hridayaayai namo Namaha

Om Satyasampurnavijnaana siddhidaayai namo Namaha

Om Shriilochanakritollasa phaladaayai namo Namaha

Om Shriisudhaabdhimanidviipa madhyagaayai namo Namaha

Om Dakshaadhvaravinirbheda saadhanaayai namo Namaha

Om Shriinaathasodariibhuuta shobhitaayai namo Namaha

Om Chandrashekharabhaktaarti bhanjanaayai namo Namaha

Om Sarvopaadhivinirmukta chaitanyaayai namo Namaha

Om Naamapaarayanaabhiishta phaladaayai namo Namaha

Om Srishtisthititirodhaana sankalpaayai namo Namaha   80

Om Shriishodashaakshariimantra madhyagaayai namo Namaha

Om Anaadyantasvayambhuuta divyamurtyai namo Namaha

Om Bhaktahansaparimukhya viyogaayai namo Namaha

Om Maatrimandalasanyukta lalitaayai namo Namaha

Om Bhandadaityamahaasattva naashanaayai namo Namaha

Om Kruurabhandashiracchheda nipunaayai namo Namaha

Om Dhaatrachyutasuraadhiisha sukhadaayai namo Namaha

Om Chandamundanishumbhaadi khandanaayai namo Namaha

Om Raktaaksharaktajihvaadi shikshanaayai namo Namaha

Om Mahishaasuradorviirya nigrahaayai namo Namaha   90

Om Abhrakeshamahotsaaha kaaranaayai namo Namaha

Om Maheshayuktanatanata tparaayai namo Namaha

Om Nijabhartrimukhaambhoja chintanaayai namo Namaha

Om Vrishabhadhvajavijnaana bhaavanaayai namo Namaha

Om Janmamrityujaraaroga bhanjanaayai namo Namaha

Om Vidheyamuktavijnana siddhidaayai namo Namaha

Om Kaamakrodhaadishadvarga naashanaayai namo Namaha

Om Raajaraajaarchitapada sarojaayai namo Namaha

Om Sarvavedaantasansiddha sutatvaayai namo Namaha   100

Om Shriiviirabhaktavijnaana vidhanaayai namo Namaha

Om Asheshadushtadanuja sudanaayai namo Namaha

Om Saakshaacchhriidakshinaamurti manojnaayai namo Namaha

Om Hayamedhaagrasampujya mahimaayai namo Namaha

Om Dakshaprajaapatisuta veshaadhyaayai namo Namaha

Om Sumabaanekshukodanda manditaayai namo Namaha

Om Nityayauvanamaangalya mangalaayai namo Namaha

Om Mahaadevasamaayukta shariiraayai namo Namaha   108

Om Mahaadevaratautsukya mahaadevyai namo Namaha

Om Chaturvimshachitatwaika shariraayai namoNamaha

Note:

- After chanting above mantras, ring the bell and show the dhoop for Goddess Lalitha. Then offer fruits or milk/ sweets to her. We can also light up ghee lamp or sesame oil lamp if required! [Or this can be done after finishing other Devi poojas & Mirthyanja pooja also]

Then next…. Gatkamaala Devi pooja starts in main kalasam vessel!….

Start offering flowers in the main kalasam itself for chanting Balambika/Gatkamala ashtothram/ other mantras…..

CHAPTER 13 – BALA THIRIPURA SUNDARI POOJA DEVI GATKAMAALA

Chant Bala Thiripura Sundari Gayatri & Moola mantra 1 time.....

Balambika Gayatri Mantra

Om Balambikaya Vithmahe; Thiripuraya Dheemihi | Dhanno Devi Prachotayad |

Shree Balambika Moola Mantra

Om Sreem; Kreem, Gleem Devi Gatkamala Ya Namaha:

Om aim hrim sreem aim klim sauhu; Om namah tripura sundari namaha:

Then Offer flowers/ Akshadha (yellow rice) in main kalasam and chant the Balambika Devi 183 names (Ashtothram plus).

Balambika/ Gatkamala Ashtothram Plus

Om	Tripura sundaryai	Namaha
Om	Hrudaya devi	Namaha
Om	Siro devī	Namaha
Om	Sikha devī	Namaha
Om	Kavacha devi	Namaha
Om	Netra devi	Namaha
Om	Astra devi	Namaha
Om	Kameswari	Namaha
Om	Bhaga mālini	Namaha
Om	Nitya klinne	Namaha
Om	Bherunde	Namaha
Om	Vahni vāsini	Namaha
Om	Mahā vajreswarī	Namaha
Om	Siva dooti	Namaha
Om	Twarite	Namaha
Om	Kula sundari	Namaha
Om	Nitye	Namaha
Om	Nīla patāke	Namaha

Om	Vijay	Namaha
Om	Sarva mangala	Namaha
Om	Jwālā mālini	Namaha
Om	Chitre	Namaha
Om	Maha nitye	Namaha
Om	Parameswara parameswari	Namaha
Om	Mitreśa mayi	Namaha
Om	Sashthisa mayi	Namaha
Om	Uddisa mayi	Namaha
Om	Charya nadha mayi	Namaha
Om	Lopā mudrā mayi	Namaha
Om	Agastya mayi	Namaha
Om	Kāla tāpana mayi	Namaha
Om	Dharma charya mayi	Namaha
Om	Mukta kesīswara mayi	Namaha
Om	Dipa kalā nādha mayi	Namaha
Om	Vishnu deva mayi	Namaha
Om	Prabhā kara deva mayi	Namaha
Om	Tejo deva mayi	Namaha
Om	Manoja deva mayi	Namaha
Om	Kalyana deva mayi	Namaha
Om	Vāsu deva mayi	Namaha
Om	Ratna deva mayi	Namaha
Om	Srī rāmānanda mayi	Namaha
Om	Anima siddhi	Namaha
Om	Laghima siddhi	Namaha
Om	Garimā siddhe	Namaha
Om	Mahima siddhi	Namaha
Om	Sarva siddhi	Namaha
Om	Vasitwa siddhe	Namaha
Om	Prākāmya siddhe	Namaha
Om	Bhukti siddhe	Namaha
Om	Ichchhā siddhe	Namaha
Om	Prapti siddhi	Namaha
Om	Sarva kama siddhi	Namaha

Om	Brahmi	Namaha
Om	Maheswari	Namaha
Om	Kaumārī	Namaha
Om	Vaishnavi	Namaha
Om	Vārāhi	Namaha
Om	Māhendri	Namaha
Om	Chāmunde	Namaha
Om	Mahā lakshmi	Namaha
Om	Sarva sankshobh	Namaha
Om	Sarva vidrāviṇi	Namaha
Om	Sarvā karshiṇi	Namaha
Om	Sarva vasankari	Namaha
Om	Sarvon mādhini	Namaha
Om	Sarva mahānkuse	Namaha
Om	Sarva khechari	Namaha
Om	Sarva bīje	Namaha
Om	Sarva yone	Namaha
Om	Sarva trikhande	Namaha
Om	Trailokya mohana chakra swāminī	Namaha
Om	Prakaṭa yogini	Namaha
Om	Kāmā karshiṇi	Namaha
Om	Buddhya karshini	Namaha
Om	Ahankārā karshiṇi	Namaha
Om	Sabdā karshiṇi	Namaha
Om	Sparsā karshiṇi	Namaha
Om	Rūpā karshiṇi	Namaha
Om	Rasā karshiṇi	Namaha
Om	Gandhā karshini	Namaha
Om	Chitta karshini	Namaha
Om	Dhairya karshini	Namaha
Om	Smrutyā karshini	Namaha
Om	Nama karshini	Namaha
Om	Bījā karshiṇi	Namaha
Om	Ātmā karshiṇi	Namaha
Om	Amrutā karshinī	Namaha

Om	Sareerā karshiṇi	Namaha
Om	Sarvasa pari puraka chakra swāminī	Namaha
Om	Gupta yogini	Namaha
Om	Ananga kusume	Namaha
Om	Ananga mekhale	Namaha
Om	Ananga madane	Namaha
Om	Ananga madanāture	Namaha
Om	Ananga rekhe	Namaha
Om	Ananga vegini	Namaha
Om	Anangānkuće	Namaha
Om	Ananga mālini	Namaha
Om	Sarva sankshobhana chakra swamini	Namaha
Om	Gupta tara yogini	Namaha
Om	Sarva sankshobhiṇi	Namaha
Om	Sarva vidrāviṇi	Namaha
Om	Sarvā karshiṇi	Namaha
Om	Sarvā hlādini	Namaha
Om	Sarva sammohini	Namaha
Om	Sarva stambhini	Namaha
Om	Sarva jhrumbhiṇi	Namaha
Om	Sarva vasankari	Namaha
Om	Sarva ranjani	Namaha
Om	Sarvon mādhini	Namaha
Om	Sarvārdha sādhike	Namaha
Om	Sarva sampatti pūraṇi	Namaha
Om	Sarva mantra mayi	Namaha
Om	Sarva dwandwa kshayankari	Namaha
Om	Sarva saubhāgya dāyaka chakra swāmini	Namaha
Om	Sampradaya yogini	Namaha
Om	Sarva siddhi prade	Namaha
Om	Sarva sampat prade	Namaha
Om	Sarva priyankari	Namaha
Om	Sarva mangala kāriṇi	Namaha
Om	Sarva kāma prade	Namaha
Om	Sarva duhkha vimochanī	Namaha

Om	Sarva mrutyu prasamanī	Namaha
Om	Sarva vighna nivāriṇi	Namaha
Om	Sarvānga sundari	Namaha
Om	Sarva saubhagya dayinī	Namaha
Om	Sarvārdha sādhaka chakra swāmini	Namaha
Om	Kulottirna yogini	Namaha
Om	Sarvajne	Namaha
Om	Sarva sakte	Namaha
Om	Sarvaiswarya pradāyini	Namaha
Om	Sarva jnāna mayi	Namaha
Om	Sarva vyādhi vināsini	Namaha
Om	Sarva dhāra swarūpe	Namaha
Om	Sarva pāpa hare	Namaha
Om	Sarvānanda mayi	Namaha
Om	Sarva rakshā swarūpiṇi	Namaha
Om	Sarvepsita phala prade	Namaha
Om	Sarva rakshākara chakra swāmini	Namaha
Om	Nigarbha yogini	Namaha
Om	Vasini	Namaha
Om	Kāmeswari	Namaha
Om	Modini	Namaha
Om	Vimale	Namaha
Om	Arune	Namaha
Om	Jayini	Namaha
Om	Sarveswari	Namaha
Om	Kaulini	Namaha
Om	Sarva roga hara chakra swamini	Namaha
Om	Rahasya yogini	Namaha
Om	Banini	Namaha
Om	Chāpini	Namaha
Om	Pasini	Namaha
Om	Ankusini	Namaha
Om	Maha kameśwarī	Namaha
Om	Maha vajreśwari	Namaha
Om	Maha bhaga mälini	Namaha

Om	Sarva siddhi prada chakra swămini	Namaha
Om	Ati rahasya yogini	Namaha
Om	Srī sri maha bhattärike	Namaha
Om	Sarvānanda maya chakra swamini	Namaha
Om	Parāpara rahasya yogini	Namaha
Om	Tripure	Namaha
Om	Tripuresi	Namaha
Om	Tripura sundari	Namaha
Om	Tripura vāsini	Namaha
Om	Tripura śrih	Namaha
Om	Tripura maalini	Namaha
Om	Tripura siddhe	Namaha
Om	Tripuramba	Namaha
Om	Mahā tripura sundari	Namaha
Om	Maha maheswarī	Namaha
Om	Maha maha rajñí	Namaha
Om	Maha maha sakte	Namaha
Om	Maha maha gupte	Namaha
Om	Mahā mahā jnapte	Namaha
Om	Maha mahanandi	Namaha
Om	Mahã maha skandhe	Namaha
Om	Maha mahaśaye	Namaha
Om	Mahā mahā Srī chakra nagara sāmrajni	Namaha
Om	Sri lalitāmbikāyai	Namaha

Namaste namaste namaste namo namaha

Note:

- After chanting above mantras, ring the bell and show the dhoop for Goddess Balambika. Then offer fruits or milk/ sweets to her. We can also light up ghee lamp or sesame oil lamp if required! [Or this can be done after finishing next Mirthyanja pooja also]

Then next.... Mirthyanja pooja starts in main kalasam vessel!....

Start offering flowers in the main kalasam itself for chanting Lord Shiva names & Mirthyanja mantras.....(simple one)

CHAPTER 14 – MAHA RUDRA - MIRTHYANJA POOJA

This Maha Mirthyanja Pooja is mainly for removal of diseases and improves longevity in general. You will get Lord Rudran (Shiva) to provide all the benefits with this mirthyanja mantra.

First of all chant the following Gayatri Mantra and Moola Mantra for Lord Shiva 1 time.

Rudra Gayatri Mantra
Om Thathpurushaya Vithmahe | Maha Devaya Dheemihi; | Dhanno Rudra Prachothayad |

Rudra Moola Mantra
Om Sreem Kreem Kleem Maha Rudraya Namaha|

Then chant the following 1 time each and offer flowers:

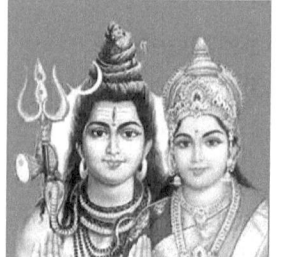

- Om Shivaya Namaha
- Om Mirthyanjaya Namaha
- Om Rudraya Namaha
- Om Neelagandaya Namaha
- Om Bhavaya Namaha
- Om Pasupathe Namaha
- Om Amrudesaya Namaha
- Om Sarvaya Namaha
- Om Mahabalaya Namaha
- Om Maheshwaraya Namaha
- Om Eswaraya Namaha
- Om Mahadevaya Namaha

Then say for yourself or others with STAR NAME, RASI NAME, GOTHRAM NAME (if known), YOUR NAME...... then followed by mirthyanja mantra to be chanted!

Example: Suppose your star is "Chithira"; rasi is "Thulam"; gothram is "Viswamithra" & your name "Anand" means, and then chant as follows.

Step 1: "Chitra nakshathra; Thula rasi jadha-sya; Viswamithra gothra-sya; Anand naama devasya",

[If you don't know other things except your name means, then say your name only and go to next step]

Step 2: "Aayul virdhi virdhiya; sarwa rogon nasaya; dhanaam virdhi virdhiya; sarwa chathroon nasaya; sarwa dhirshti nasaya",

Step 3:

"OM THRIYAMBAGAM YOJAMAGE SUGANDHIM BUSTIVARDHANAM; URUVARUGA BANDHANADH MIRTHYOR MOOSHIYA MAAMARTHAADH SWAHA:"

Offer flowers on Kalasam. Then again repeat above steps atleast for 10 times. Some people will do 16 or 28 or 32 or 54 or 108 also.

The above mantra is called mirthyanja mantra and very powerful to keep a person with healthy life and prosperity.

Note:

- After chanting above mantras atleast for 10 times, ring the bell and show the dhoop for all god/goddess together. Then offer fruits or milk/ sweets. We can also light up ghee lamp or sesame oil lamp if required! (mandatory).

Say "Dhoopam Samarpayami", "Dheepam Samarpayami", Thambula Neivedhyam Samarpayami", "Sarva Ubachaaran Samarpayami"! "Aachamaneeyam Samarpayami"|

Sprinkle water from bowl or glass with hand and put some flowers after showing lamp.

****

Then next….one is Nagaraja Swami pooja useful for kala sarpa dhosham or naga dhosham …..starts in main kalasam vessel!….

Start offering flowers in the main kalasam itself for chanting Nagaraja ashtothram/ other mantras…..

CHAPTER 15 – NAGARAJA SWAMI POOJA

Chant the following Nagaraja Gayatri mantra and Moola mantra 1 time....each.

Nagaraja Gayatri Mantra:
OM NAGARAJAYA VITHMAHE | SARPARAJAYA DHEEMIHI | DHANNO AADHISHESHA PRACHOTHAYAD |

Nagaraja Moola Mantra:
Om Sreem Kreem Kleem Nagarajaya Namaha:

Nagaraja Swami Ashtothram Namavali (108 Names)
Om anantaay Namaha
Om vaasudevaakhyaay Namaha
Om takshakaay Namaha
Om vishvatOmukhaay Namaha
Om kaarkotakaay Namaha
Om mahaapadmaay Namaha
Om padmaay Namaha
Om shankhaay Namaha
Om shivapriyaay Namaha
Om dhrtaraashtraay Namaha
Om shankhapaalaay Namaha
Om gulikaay Namaha
Om ishtadaayine Namaha
Om naagaraajaay Namaha
Om puraanapurooshaay Namaha   15

Om anaghaay Namaha
Om vishvaroopaay Namaha
Om maheedhaarine Namaha
Om kaamadaayine Namaha
Om suraarchitaay Namaha
Om kundaprabhaay Namaha
Om bahushirase Namaha
Om dakshaay Namaha
Om daamodaraay Namaha
Om aksharaay Namaha

Om ganaadhipaay Namaha
Om mahaasenaay Namaha
Om punyamoortaye Namaha
Om ganapriyaay Namaha
Om varapradaay Namaha   30

Om vaayubhakshaay Namaha
Om vishvadhaarine Namaha
Om vihangamaay Namaha
Om putrapradaay Namaha
Om punyaroopaay Namaha
Om pannageshaay Namaha
Om bileshayaay Namaha
Om parameshthine Namaha
Om pashupataye Namaha
Om pavanaashine Namaha
Om balapradaay Namaha
Om daityahantre Namaha
Om dayaaroopaay Namaha
Om dhanapradaay Namaha
Om matidaayine Namaha   45

Om mahaamaayine Namaha
Om madhuvairine Namaha
Om mahoragaay Namaha
Om bhujageshaay Namaha
Om bhoOmaroopaay Namaha
Om bheemakaayaay Namaha
Om bhayaapahrte Namaha
Om shuklaroopaay Namaha
Om shuddhadehaay Namaha
Om shokahaarine Namaha
Om shubhapradaay Namaha
Om santaanadaayine Namaha
Om sarpeshaay Namaha
Om sarvadaayine Namaha
Om sareesrpaay Namaha   60

Om lakshmeekaraay Namaha
Om laabhadaayine Namaha

Om lalitaay Namaha
Om lakshmanaakrtaye Namaha
Om dayaaraashaye Namaha
Om daasharathaye Namaha
Om damaashrayaay Namaha
Om ramyaroopaay Namaha
Om raamabhaktaay Namaha
Om ranadheeraay Namaha
Om ratipradaay Namaha
Om saumitraye Namaha
Om somasankaashaay Namaha
Om sarparaajaay Namaha
Om sataampriyaay Namaha   75

Om karburaay Namaha
Om kaamyaphaladaay Namaha
Om kireetine Namaha
Om kinnaraarchitaay Namaha
Om paataalavaasine Namaha
Om paramaay Namaha
Om phanaamandalamanditaay Namaha
Om baahuleyaay Namaha
Om bhaktanidhaye Namaha
Om bhoomidhaarine Namaha
Om bhavapriyaay Namaha
Om naaraayanaay Namaha
Om naanaaroopaay Namaha
Om natapriyaay Namaha
Om kaakodaraay Namaha   90

Om kaamyaroopaay Namaha
Om kalyaanaay Namaha
Om kaamitaarthadaay Namaha
Om hataasuraay Namaha
Om halyaheenaay Namaha
Om harshadaay Namaha
Om harabhooshanaay Namaha
Om jagadaadaye Namaha
Om jaraaheenaay Namaha
Om jaatishoonyaay Namaha

Om jaganmayaay Namaha
Om vandhyaatvadoshashamanaay Namaha
Om varaputraphalapradaay Namaha
Om balabhadraroopaay Namaha
Om shreekrshnapoorvajaay Namaha
Om vishnutalpaay Namaha
Om balvaladhnaay Namaha
Om bhoodharaay Namaha   108

Note:

- After chanting above mantras, ring the bell and show the dhoop for Nagaraja Swami. Then offer fruits or milk/ sweets to her. We can also light up ghee lamp or sesame oil lamp if required! (optional).

Next is... Murugan (Subramanya Swami) pooja for mainly Manglik (Chevvai or Angaraga Dhosham remedy). Finishing with Subramanya Swami pooja and after this finally also you can show dhoop, deepam, prasadam or other offerings....

CHAPTER 16 – SUBRAMANYA SWAMI POOJA

Chant the following murugan/ subramanya Gayatri mantra and Moola mantra 1 time….each.

Subramanya Gayatri Mantra:
OM THATH-PURUSHAYA VITHMAHE | MAHA-SENAAYA DHEEMIHI | DHANNO SHANMUGA PRACHOTHAYAD |

Chatru Samhara Moola Mantra:
OM CHATRU SAMHARA; SADAAKSHARA, ASTHRAAYA BHAT SWAHA:

Offer flowers or yellow rice in main kalasam vessel and chant the following ashtothram 108 names….

Subramanya Swami Ashtothram Namavali

Om Skandaya Namaha

Om Guhaya Namaha

Om Shanmuga Namaha

Om Phalanetrasutaya Namaha

Om Prabhave Namaha

Om Pingalaya Namaha

Om Kritikasunave Namaha

Om Sikivahaya Namaha

Om Dvisadbhujaya Namaha

Om Dvisannetraya Namaha

Om Saktidharaya Namaha

Om Pisitasaprabhamjanaya Namaha

Om Tarakasurasamharine Namaha

Om Raksobalavimardhanaya Namaha

Om Mattaya Namaha

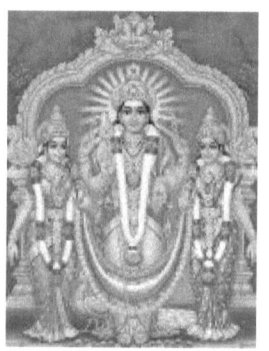

15

Om Pramattaya Namaha

Om Unmattaya Namaha

Om Surasainyasuraksakaya Namaha

Om Ganapataye Namaha

Om Prajnaya Namaha

Om Krpalave Namaha

Om Bhaktavatsalaya Namaha

Om Umasutaya Namaha

Om Saktidharaya Namaha

Om Kumaraya Namaha

Om Kraunchadharanaya Namaha

Om Senanyai Namaha

Om Agnijanmane Namaha

Om Visakhaya Namaha

Om Sankaratmajaya Namaha   30

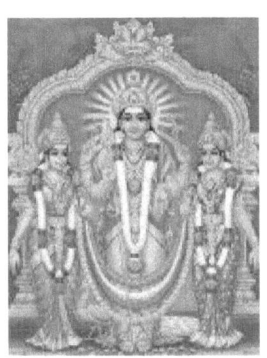

Om Sivasvamine Namaha

Om Sainathaya Namaha

Om Sarvasvamine Namaha

Om Sanatanaya Namaha

Om Anantasaktaye Namaha

Om Akshobhya Namaha

Om Parvatipriyanandanaya Namaha

Om Gangasutaya Namaha

Om Sarodbhutaya Namaha

Om Pavakatmajaya Namaha

Om Ganasvamine Namaha

Om Atmabhuve Namaha

Om Jrmbhaya Namaha

Om Prajrmbhaya Namaha

Om Ujjrmbhaya Namaha   45

Om Kamalasanasamstutaya Namaha

Om Ekavarnaya Namaha

Om Dvivarnaya Namaha

Om Trivarnaya Namaha

Om Sumanoharaya Namaha

Om Chaturvarnaya Namaha

Om Panchavarnaya Namaha

Om Prajapataye Namaha

Om Ganapataye Namaha

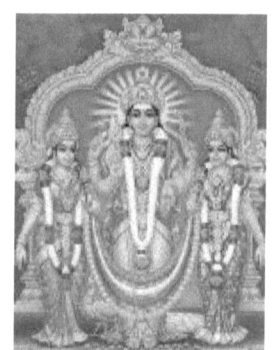

Om Agnigarbhaya Namaha

Om Samigarbhaya Namaha

Om Visvaretase Namaha

Om Surarighnaya Namaha

Om Harodvarnaya Namaha

Om Bhaskaraya Namah   60

Om Vasavaya Namaha

Om Vatuvesabhrte Namaha

Om Pusne Namaha

Om Gabhastine Namaha

Om Gahanaya Namaha

Om Chandravarnaya Namaha

Om Kaladharaya Namaha

Om Mayadharaya Namaha

Om Mahamayine Namaha

Om Kaivalyaya Namaha

Om Sakalatmakaya Namaha

Om Visvayonaye Namaha

Om Ameyatmane Namaha

Om Tejonidhaye Namaha

Om Anamayaya Namaha   75

Om Paramesthine Namaha

Om Parabrahmane Namaha

Om Vedagharbayanamah

Om Viradvapusenamah

Om Pulindakanyabharte Namaha

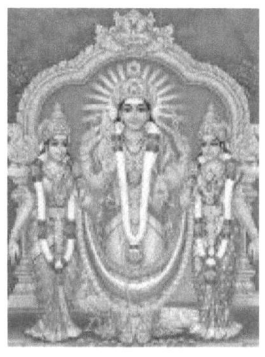

Om Mahasarasvatavrtaya Namaha

Om Asritakhiladatre Namaha

Om Choraghnaya Namaha

Om Roganasanaya Namaha

Om Ananda Murtaye Namaha

Om Anandaya Namaha

Om Sikhandikrtaketanaya Namaha

Om Dhambhaya Namaha

Om Paramadhambhaya Namaha

Om Mahadhambaya Namaha   90

Om Vrsakapaye Namaha

Om Karanopattadehaya Namaha

Om Karanatitavigrahaya Namaha

Om Anisvaraya Namaha

Om Amrtaya Namaha

Om Pranaya Namaha

Om Pranayama Narayanaya Namaha

Om Viruddhahantre Namaha

Om Viraghnaya Namaha

Om Raktasyamagalaya Namaha

Om Mahate Namaha

Om Subrahmanyaya Namaha

Om Guhaya Namaha

Om Brahmanyaya Namaha

Om Vamsayrddhikaraya Namaha

Om Brahmanapriyaya Namaha

Om Aksayaphalapradaya Namaha

Om Vedavedhyaya Namaha   108

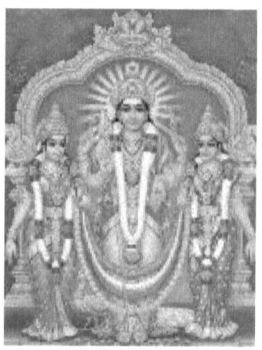

Note:

- After chanting above mantras, ring the bell and show the dhoop for all god/goddess together. Then offer fruits or milk/ sweets. We can also light up ghee lamp or sesame oil lamp if required! (mandatory).

Say "Dhoopam Samarpayami", "Dheepam Samarpayami", Thambula Neivedhyam Samarpayami", "Sarva Ubachaaran Samarpayami"!,......Sprinkle water from bowl or glass with hand and put some flowers after showing lamp. Do full namaskaaram on the floor 2 or 4 times and pray well. Entire parigaram pooja is over!

****

POOJA/ WORSHIP CONCLUSION

➤ The entire 16 chapters are covering very powerful pooja with 7 Goddesses, Ganapathy-Hanuman, Navagraga, Nagaraja and Subramanya Swami. This is the best remedy pooja for anything.

➤ As we perform 7 Devis' pooja in the remedy; it is also called Saptha Kaali Pooja.

➤ The poojas can be done simply with idol/image or 1 kalasam vessel/ or with decorated things like 2 or 3 kalasams together; but mainly our intention and bakthi is very important to get divine blessings for any purpose.

➤ Mostly all the Sanskrit words are in English; you can also refer other online resources. Easy to chant and do the poojas.

➤ Sample pooja pictures are given in forst 2 chapters.

➤ You can do the poojas your own with ablution with clean mind and place.

➤ A guruji or elders or experienced people can also help you to do this if you are willing to do so.

➤ For most of the remedies, all the above poojas are enough.

➤ After pooja worship; you can use the kalasam water to take bath and sprinkle at home in and around for purification.

➤ Additionally "Additional Chapter - Homam/ Havan/ Yagnam" is given in the next chapter for extended pooja homam. Will be useful to perform homam after doing above poojas.

➤ For example, some people would be willing to do Ganapathy, Hanuman, Lakshmi and Navgraga Homam. For them, they can do those 4 poojas from the above chapters with setup and sangalpam and then extended to homam. [This is also performed in Graha Pravesam – House Warming].

➤ Anyone can split and do like this if you are willing to perform with limited poojas and homam/yagam/yagnam.

For any feedback, query or suggestions please mail to astronara@gmail.com or info@zodiacservices.net.

You can also contact via www.zodiacservices.net/contact.

THANK YOU!

Agni Hothram (Do it yourself)!

This is a kind of simple and effective method of invocation in fire to keep us healthy and wealthy. Can be performed during sun raise and (or) sun set time exactly; because of attracting good prana sakthi (pranic healing power) and divine blessings. Anyone can perform this after getting Guru upadesam (learn from Guru) simply at home with little or less mantras (chanting)

Requirements: (i) Brass/ Copper pyramid (hollow - Or check in above picture); this can be tilted and kept on a stand which is fire proof or keep on two stones. (ii) Pure cow ghee (some 30 or 50 ml) for each session. (iii) Cow dung - dried one available in alternative medical shop. or we can collect & dry it off and store. (iv) Camphor and match box or lighter. (v) Raw rice some 100 grams.

Procedure: Mix raw rice with little ghee and keep them separately. Arrange Havan kundam (Hallow prymid) on the stand or stone and load little with dried Cow dung (Gow Sanam). Light up fire on that and let it grow for few seconds.

Then add rice and ghee slowly in fire with spoon by chanting the mantras:

If morning then, **"Om Asmin Agni Kam Ganapathiye Swaha!"** - 10 times or **"Om Maha Ganapathiye Swaha"** - 10 times

Then **"Suryaya Swaha; Suryaya Idham Namaha"** - 10 times

After that **"Prajapathiye Swaha; Prajapathiye Idham Namaha"** - 10 times

Same procedure can be followed in the evening also; but instead of

Then **"Suryaya Swaha; Suryaya Idham Namaha"** - you have to chant and add ghee and rice with this mantra

Then **"Agniye Swaha; Agniye Idham Namaha"** - 10 times

Finish the Homam or Agni Hothram until Ghee and Rice are over and Say **"Sarvam Sri Krishnar-panam"** - 3 times

- Perform this at home whenever possible as it purifies air/environment, removes toxins and cure diseases etc.

- Store the ashes of this and it is amazing cure for any diseases / problems.

- For example, if you have skin problems; just apply on the same and gets cleared in few days. For any internal problems, little can be consumed with honey or water and the same will be cured. Mix little ash in water and take bath and it cleanses the whole body; and so on.

This agni-hotram can be extended to normal or detailed homam/ yagam. [Actually the Agni Hotram is not necessary!]

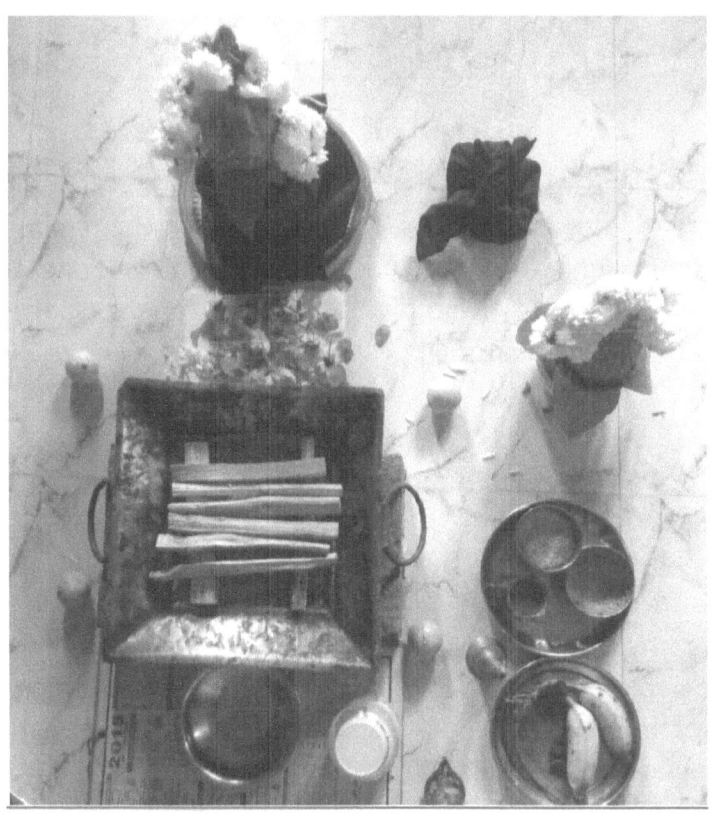

Kalasam/ Kumbam can be kept to do pooja or rituals initially using flowers or yellow rice (akshatha). Then the homam or yagam can be started using gayatri / moola mantras. Same like other previous poojas.

- <u>In General</u>: Like other poojas & worship; Homam/Yagnam can bring more cosmic energy vibrations, blessings and purification of energies in and around a particular permisis/ cure any diseases due to the effect of mantras, herbs added in fire & divine blessings.

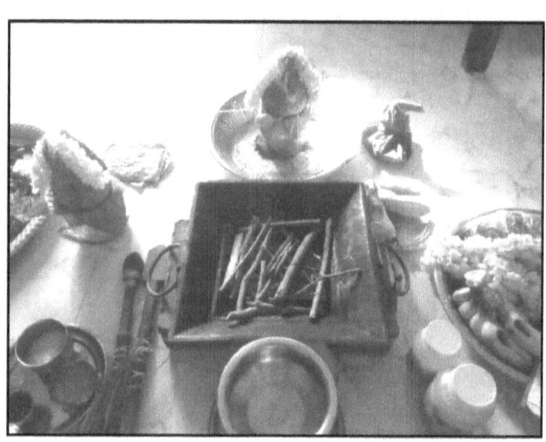

- Homam cleanses and revitalizes the environment by inflow of life-force into the atmosphere. All the people who are performing, attending and living nearby where the homam done are getting benefits improving health, wealth, destroying bad effect of evil forces (including back magic attack), abundance and prosperity etc.

- Also you can find out which is your favorable angelic assistance to worship regularly with Yantra and Mantra upadesam (method to follow) to overcome all the obstacles and improve in all the areas though the time is very bad!

- <u>Ganapathy Pooja OR Homam</u> - Must be performed before any other pooja or homam as well. Brings complete blessings of Maha Ganapathy. Basically eliminates all the obstacles, negative effect/ negative energy patterns in a place or building etc; Cures common diseases like head ache, Stomach problems, physical pain, viral fever, and so on. Good for education, house warming, prosperity, abundance, happiness, health, wealth, Navagraga dhosha/ Gajendra dhosha nivarthy.

Set up a brass havan vessel as described in the previous chapter. Or simply using bricks or stones also can be kept to form havan kundam (actual fire buring pit). Check the earlier picture. Keep some bowl for ghee to be poured for homam and two spoons to do this.

Keep thambulam (betel leaves and supari), bananas, flowers, lemons, turmeric powder, kumkum and holy rice (yellow rice mixed with turmeric powder), lamp and samith (firewoods of banian tree or jack tree etc) or herbs as required. [Shown in the next picture].

After steeing the kalasam / Kumbam vessel with water or coconut; decorate the same with flower and apply chandan kumkum. Keep a side.

Set up the havan / homam vessel with initial firewoods kept inside. Keep the ghee ready. Also, little water is taken to sprinkle - then and there in the pooja time.

Keep one Lord Ganesh / Ganapathy picture or Idol next to havan vessel for pooja. Sometimes without Kumbam or kalasam also the pooja can be performed only with idol or picture for simple pooja as per your wish.

As described in the earlier chapter that how to perform the Ganapathy pooja, please do so with 108 names, Ganapathy upanishid or 1000 names of Ganapathy etc for idol or picture or Kalasa Kumbam as per your wish.

Then start the homam (fire ritual) with ghee as described in the previous chapter (Agni Hotram).

Do all these things with holy wash or ablution with proper sangalpam or intention to get success. [Refer sangalpam in first two chapters]

Start the homam with,

Lighting up a small camphour or buring fire from match sticks, will ignite the fire. [There are some electric / electronic havan vessel also available. Please check online and buy if required].

Chant:
Asmin agni mandale' maha ganapathim aavagayami! – 1 time. (put holy rice/ yellow rice on everything)

Asmin agniye' kam ganapathiye' swaha – 3 times by pouring little drop of ghee in the fire.

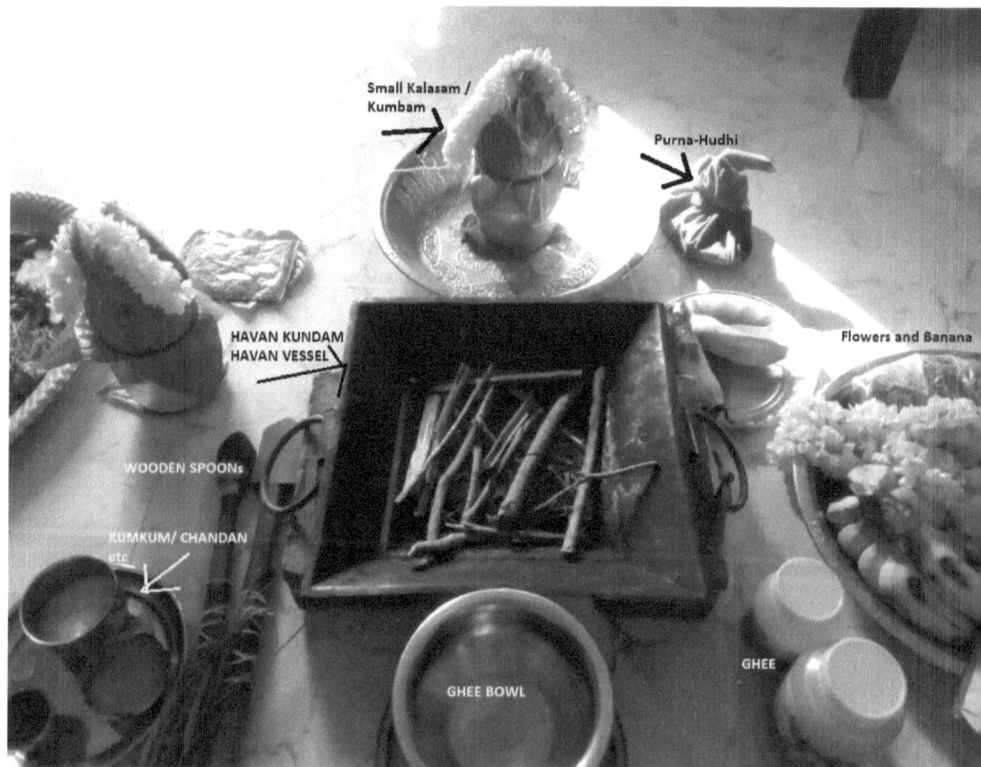

- *Ganaa naam thva ganapathikum aavamage' kaveem kaveenam upamastha vasthramam; jeyshta rajam brahmanaam; brahmanas wana aana seervana sasanam!* – *1 time* [Lord Ganesh mula mantra]

- *Om shreem hreem kleem kloum kam ganapathaye; Varavarada sarva janamme vasamaanaya swaha : - 1 time*
  [Lord Ganesh mula mantra]......given in previous pooja chapters also.
  Chant gayatri mantra 1 time and moola mantra 1 time...finally add the word "swaha" with moola mantra and pour the ghee/ put herbals in fire.

Then pour the drops of ghee one time in fire. Like wise repeat for 16 or 28 or 36 or 54 or 108 times.

[Another method is chant 108 names names from the previous chapters with "Swaha" as suffix on each name and pour drops of ghee in the fire. Example: Om Vinayagaya Swaha, Om Vigna Rajaya Swaha,...etc]

By finishing this; the actual lagu - Ganapathy homam is over.

This homam can be extended to other deities/ god/ goddess as well.

After finishing Ganapathy, do Lakshmi homam/yagnam like;

> *Chant gayatri mantra 1 time and moola mantra 1 time...finally add the word "swaha" with moola mantra and pour the ghee/ put herbals in fire.*

Chant Lakshmi Gayatri

Om Mahadevi cha vithmahe | Vishnu pathni cha dheemihi | Dhanno Lakshmi Prachothayad| 1 time

MahaLakshmi Moola mantra

Om Sreem Kreem Kleem Maha Lakshmiye Swaha: 1 time (pour ghee or put herbal in fire]

Do minimum 16 times of gayatri and moola mantra homam.
Can be done for all deities like this by referring gayatri and moola mantras from previous chapters.

After finishing all the homam whatever the god/goddess you want, then few other formalities are as follows.

Before doing any other homam, Lord Ganapathy homam is mandatory.

There is a procedure called **Purna Hudhi**; offer some food to Lord Ganesh. Just tie 2 bananas, betel leaves and supari, little coconut pieces, cashwes, dry grapes etc can be added in bundle and then offer in the fire. [if not possible, please offer only fruits like banana or apple or orange etc…stand and do]

The mantra to offer this is:

Om Purna hudhi muthamam juhodhi; sarvam vai purna hudhi:
Sarvame vapnodhi, adho iyam vai purna hudhi:
Asyameva pradhi Dhishtathi! – 1 time
[and]
Om Namo Vradha Pathaye Namo Ganapathaye' Namaha: Pramadha
Pathaye' Namasthesthu Lambodharaya; Eka Thandhaya Vigna
Vinasine, Siva Sudhaya Varadha Murthiye' Namo Namaha! – 1 time

Then put the bundled offering item as said above; slowly in the fire by praying Lord Ganesh to give us all the success in life and work. Use the holy wooden spoons to hold and put in the fire.

After that; sprinkle some water on everything and show dhoop and ghee lamp or camphour.
Then **bhali** procedure to be completed to remove evil effect during pooja or homam if any. Take two lemons and cut into four pieces. Touch in the kumkum to make it reddish and keep in the four courners of fire base outside [in clock wise direction from north east].

Mantra for this is:

Maano Mahantha Mutha Maano; Arpagam maana ushantha mutha
maa.. Ushitham Maanovathi:
Pitharam Motha Maadharam priya Maanasthanvo rudhra reerisha:
Shekthra baalaya balim thadhami! – 1 time

Then sprinkle some water on those four corners.

Then say "*Yadhasthaanam pradhishta bayaami!*" – 1 time.

Then add ghee to fire and chant;
Om Bu: swaha – Agniye idham namaha!
Om Buva swaha – Vayuve idham namaha!
Om Swa: Swaha – Suryaya idham namaha!
Om Burbuvasva – Swaha Pracha pathaye idham namaha! – 1 time

Then again add ghee and say!

Om Burbuvasva – Swaha Pracha pathaye idham namaha!
Sri Vishnave swaha; vishnave idham namaha!
Namo rudhraya pasupathaye swaha; pasupathaye idham namaha! –
1 time!

Then wash hands and sprinkle water on the divine / holy items etc.

Generally the holy spoons are tied with mango leaves or betel leaves to make it divine instruments. Those leaves can be removed and added to fire as well. Or generally take two betel leaves or holi grass and just dip in ghee and then chant: [stand and do]

Sapthathe' agne' samitha: Saptha Jikhwa,
Saptha rishiya, saptha thaama priya ni!
Saptha gothra, saptha thaathva jayathi!
Saptha yonira prunaswa kruthena swaha:
Agnaye sapthathe' idham namaha! – 1 time

Add ghee and leave the leaves into the fire. Sprinkle water and sit.

Then take little water in fingers and chant,
Adhi dhenva makstha – sprinkle right side of agni/ fire.
Anupa thenva makstha – sprinkle upside (sky)
Saraswa thenva makstha – sprinkle left side of agni/ fire.
Dheva savitha prasaavi – sprinkle clockwise of agni / fire vessel.

Then chant the following to pray god to excuse our mistakes during the pooja or homam.

Agnaye namaha: Mantra heenam, kriya heenam, bakthi heenam hudhasanaha; Yath hudham thu maya deva pari purnam thadhasthudhe'

Praaya chithaanya seshaani thapaha! Karmath magaani vai yaani sheshaama sheshaanam:
Krushnaanu smaranam, padham sri Krishna krishaha: - 1 time

Sometimes, the holy ash can be taken to add with little ghee for applying on the forehead like bindhi or kumkum. Say *"Raksha Raksha raksha"* – 1 time and apply the same.

Then sprinkle water right side with little turmeric rice.

Finally chant the following [optional]

Kaayena vaacha, manasentharyai va! Budhyath manavaa prakrudhe swabaavath! Karomi yath sagalam parasmai, naarayana yedhi samarpayami! Sarvam sri krishnarpana masthu! – 1 time.

Then sprinkle water right side and get up from homam.

- But Hanuman or Varahi or any other deity homam can be extended after Maha Ganapathy homam & purna hudhi stage as described before. That means once we finish Ganapathy homam and purna hudhi procedure as said above, we have to show dhoop, dheep and offer fruits etc, then immediately we can start hanuman or varahi homam by pouring ghee drops into fire for 16 or 28 / 108 mula mantras. Then finally we can do other procedures like Bali etc.

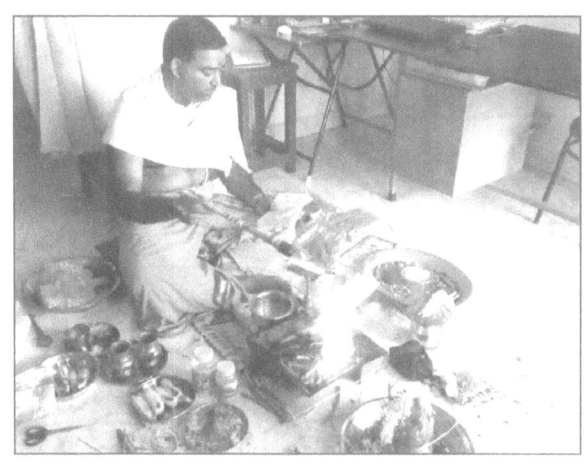

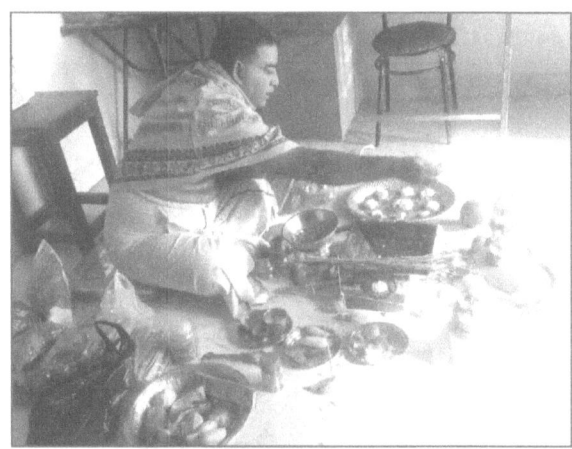

OM THATH SATH!

or any feedback, query or suggestions please mail to astronara@gmail.com or nfo@zodiacservices.net.

ou can also contact via www.zodiacservices.net/contact.

THANK YOU!

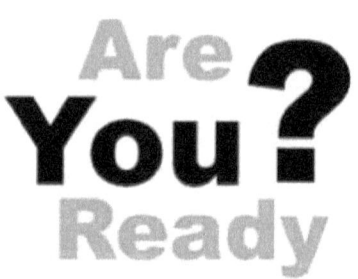

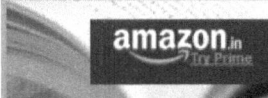

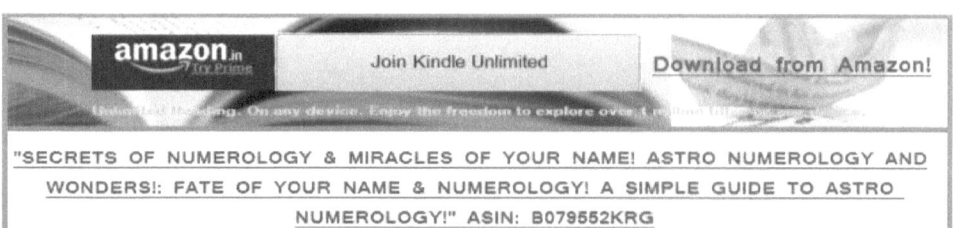